Psychology Revivals

Colour-Blindness

Originally published in 1925, this book embodies the results of research on red-green colour-blind subjects, supplemented by brief accounts of blue-yellow, total, and acquired colour-blindness to complete the description of the different forms of the defect. After a historical survey of previous work by such men as Dalton, Helmholtz, Rayleigh, Edridge-Green and others, the author deals with the most important theories of colour-blindness, and with a description of the tests and a discussion of their results.

Colour-Blindness

With a comparison of different methods of
testing colour-blindness

Mary Collins

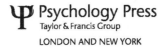

Psychology Press
Taylor & Francis Group
LONDON AND NEW YORK

First published in 1925
by Kegan Paul, Trench, Trubner & Co. Ltd

This edition first published in 2015 by Psychology Press
27 Church Road, Hove, BN3 2FA

and by Psychology Press
711 Third Avenue, New York, NY 10017

Psychology Press is an imprint of the Taylor & Francis Group, an informa business

© 1925 Mary Collins

Publisher's Note
The publisher has gone to great lengths to ensure the quality of this reprint but
points out that some imperfections in the original copies may be apparent.

Disclaimer
The publisher has made every effort to trace copyright holders and welcomes
correspondence from those they have been unable to contact.

A Library of Congress record exists under LCCN: 25012762

ISBN: 978-1-138-95305-5 (hbk)
ISBN: 978-1-315-66747-8 (ebk)
ISBN: 978-1-138-95311-6 (pbk)

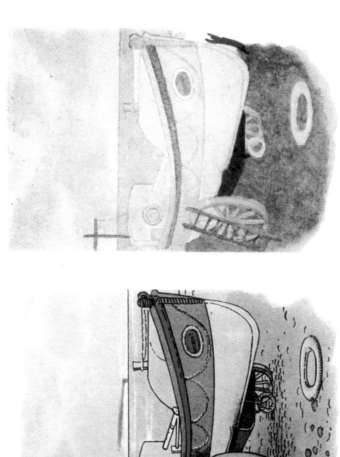

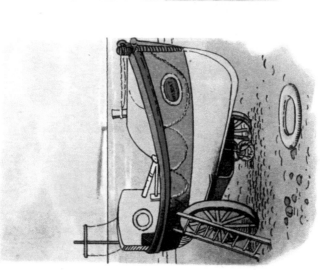

Reproduction of Picture by J. showing characteristic confusions. The red splash at the right hand side was judged to be too dark to represent the beach, so green was substituted as it was of a lighter shade of the *same* colour, and in consequence gave a more satisfactory match see p. 182).

Colour-Blindness

With a Comparison of Different Methods of Testing
Colour-Blindness

BY

MARY COLLINS

M.A., B.Ed., Ph.D.

Lecturer on Applied Psychology, Edinburgh University

With an Introduction by

DR JAMES DREVER,

George Combe Department of Psychology, Edinburgh University

LONDON

KEGAN PAUL, TRENCH, TRUBNER & CO., LTD.

NEW YORK: HARCOURT, BRACE & COMPANY, INC.

1925

Printed in Great Britain by
MACKAYS   LTD.,   CHATHAM

CONTENTS

v

CONTENTS

PREFACE

THIS book embodies the results of research on red-green colour-blind subjects, supplemented by brief accounts of blue-yellow, total, and acquired colour-blindness to complete the description of the different forms of the defect.

The tests on the colour-blinds were carried out unbiased by any preconceived theory and no rigid classification was attempted during the experiments themselves. As the investigation proceeded, the facts obtained gradually centred round many of the characteristics peculiar to the colour-blind. The subjects were ten in all: eight of them were students attending the graduating course in Experimental Psychology, the other two were science students. All, therefore, were accustomed to experimental procedure, and may be regarded as reliable subjects. I should like here to express my gratitude to them for the many hours which they placed at my disposal, and for their very helpful co-operation.

The experiments were carried out at different hours in the George Combe Psychological Laboratory. The periods of testing lasted one hour at a time with rest intervals, and as far as possible fatigue was avoided. The subjects are all cases of congenital dichromasy, and suffer from the most common form of this defect—an inability to distinguish red and green.

I have been rather fortunate in testing subjects whose respective colour defects show differences in degree. At first, it was puzzling to explain why, for example, in colour-matching, an equation could be obtained with one subject and not with a second. Then, as the facts accumulated, the explanation stood out clearly that the subjects were not all suffering from total blindness to red and green, but that in their inability to discern these colours they could be graded as in a scale. This result appears to me a conclusive one, and it was verified repeatedly.

One other interesting result which emerged from the tests was the indication of the existence of two neutral bands—one in the blue-green region of the spectrum, the other beyond the spectrum, in the complementary purple. This fact was established by more than one test, but first came to light when employing the Bradley Paper Test. The presence of both bands was definitely established in the case of some of the subjects, and was certainly indicated in others. This finding serves to explain some of the confusions made by colour-blinds, and it has also an important theoretical bearing. Further, cases of shortening of the violet end of the spectrum may not be so unusual—for it seems probable that the shortening may be explained by the extension of the second neutral band into the violet region, thereby causing a cutting-off of the violet rays.

This investigation is merely an attempt to clear up some of the problems which have gathered round the vastly interesting condition of colour-blindness.

I should like to express my indebtedness to Dr Drever for his invaluable assistance and encouragement throughout the investigation, and for his help in preparing the book for the Press. My thanks are due to Professor Roaf for allowing me to incorporate his test ; also, acknowledgment must be made of the courtesy of the Royal Society of Edinburgh in granting me permission to reproduce FIGS. VIII and IX from their *Transactions*.

M.C.

The University,
  Edinburgh.

INTRODUCTION

In the present study of colour-blindness by Dr Mary Collins are given the results of an investigation begun some four years ago in the George Combe Psychological Laboratory at Edinburgh. The beginnings of the investigation were small and unpretentious. Students, who had difficulty with some of the colour experiments in the laboratory, were tested with Stilling's Tables. In the class of the year referred to no fewer than ten students were found, who failed to such an extent with this test as to be considered for practical purposes as colour-blind. The fact that so large a number of colour-blind subjects was available suggested the further exploration of their colour experience, with such tests as were to hand in the laboratory. Dr Collins undertook this exploration, and as it soon became evident that results of considerable psychological interest were being obtained, the investigation was gradually extended until it reached the dimensions indicated by the book before us.

Ostensibly the main object of the wider investigation was a comparison with respect to efficiency of various tests that had at different times been suggested and employed for the diagnosis of colour defect. The practical value of such a comparison is more or less obvious, and this practical value has been kept in view throughout, and, as will be seen, largely determines the order of presentation. But the practical value begins and ends with a comparison of the various tests and methods with respect to their facility in use and the efficiency with which they bring out colour defect. The facts relating to the colour-vision of the colour-blind, which throw light on the nature of the colour experience of the colour-blind, are, as it were, by-products of the experiments, but nevertheless these are the centre of psychological interest, and, one might also say, of general interest. On these the book bases its claim to the attention of a wider circle of readers than those who are merely concerned with the practical use of tests for colour-blindness.

As Dr Collins has pointed out, the curious and interesting phenomena associated with the condition commonly designated colour-blindness do not appear to have attracted sustained and systematic attention on the part of the scientist until comparatively modern times. Perhaps we ought not to be surprised at this when we remember that many colour-blinds remain ignorant of their own defect, or at least of its real nature. Of course, it is impossible to compare directly one individual's sensation, say, of red, with that of another individual. So long as they both call the same things red, they can have no reason to suppose that their experiences of red are different. Hence, if, as sometimes happens, the colour-blind individual finds that for the most part he calls the same things red as other people call red, even though he does not know what it is to experience red, he will have no reason to suppose that his colour vision is different from that of other people. When, however, the colour defect is extreme, strange things cannot help happening. A speaker—obviously a typical red-green blind—at the Liverpool meeting of the British Association in 1923, describing his own experiences, said that he could see unripe strawberries in his garden, but he could never see ripe strawberries. Dr George Wilson[1] gives

---

[1] Researches on Colour-Blindness, 1855.

numerous instances of a similar kind, illustrating the interesting, and often amusing, results in behaviour, which an inability of this kind may occasionally involve. Thus he relates how an undertaker on one occasion covered a coffin with bright red in place of black, how a doctor stated that he had never met with a case of scarlet fever in his practice, and how a gentleman, meeting a lady dressed in green, thought she was in mourning and offered his condolences. Such striking manifestations of colour defect could hardly fail to excite at least transient curiosity and amusement, but the curiosity did not take on a scientific complexion till Dalton, the famous chemist, undertook the investigation of the phenomena of colour defect in his own case.

Once scientific thought was directed systematically to the phenomena of colour-blindness, their important bearing on theories of colour vision became immediately obvious, and this has ever since been the main interest stimulating and guiding scientific study of the phenomena. Theories of colour vision were, of course, in existence long before this scientific study of the phenomena of colour-blindness began. Such theories date from the time of the Greeks. There were even psychological, as distinct from physical, theories from comparatively early times. As early as the beginning of the sixteenth century Leonardo da Vinci had formulated on a psychological basis a four-colour theory, which anticipated the well-known colour theory developed by Goethe, both with respect to conclusions and with respect to supporting arguments, and which, as far as it went, was almost identical with the theory now associated with the name of the German physiologist Hering. But although psychological or physiological theories were in existence when the phenomena of colour-blindness began to receive systematic attention from the scientist, the great majority of colour theories were definitely physical, and these physical colour theories formed the mental background against which the facts of colour-blindness came to be projected, the apperception-mass which was active in their interpretation.

Dr Collins does well to call attention to the result of this state of matters on the study of the actual phenomena. When, on my suggestion, she undertook a purely psychological, and as far as possible unbiased, investigation of the facts, I was myself an adherent of the Hering theory —a physiological or psychological theory—and I was half amused and half irritated by the obstinacy with which she refused to accept my interpretations, or at least to allow her experiments to be controlled by my theory. She was determined to be free from a bias in the direction of a psychological no less than of a physical theory. It is not too much to say that her attitude has been entirely justified by the results. In any case it was unquestionably the true scientific attitude.

This question of psychological or physical theories of colour-vision is of some importance. It is clear that colour-vision is primarily the field of the psychologist. This should only require to be stated in order to be universally accepted. The phenomena are no doubt of interest to the worker in the field of physical optics, but they are in themselves psychological phenomena, and to regard them in any other way is thoroughly unscientific. After the psychologist the physiologist is next concerned. He also must be allowed his say before the problems really become problems for the physicist.

It must not be imagined that the interest of this contention is purely academic. A single illustration will suffice to show how fundamental it is. For the physicist the colours seen by the eye of the human being do not represent the starting-point of investigation. For him colours present themselves as a continuous rectilinear series, extending from red at the one end to violet at the other, and corresponding to ethereal vibrations of different wave-lengths. This series is but a part of a physical series, the other parts of which—at the two extremes— are invisible to the human eye. Red and violet are as far distant from one another as they could be, representing respectively the two extremes of the visible series. When we pass beyond violet, we still get the physical series, but the more rapid ethereal vibrations are not visible ; similarly, when we pass beyond red, we get to invisible ethereal vibrations once more, but with slower vibration rate. From our present point of view, the main facts are : that the series is rectilinear and continuous, and that red and violet are remote from one another.

Now the facts of colour-vision for physiologist and psychologist are quite different. In the first place the series of colours is circular, not rectilinear, red and violet approaching one another, and the gap between being bridged by the purples. In the second place there is a certain characteristic lack of continuity. Certain colours appear psychologically primitive, pure, or separate, others, on the contrary, presenting themselves as more or less mixed. Thus red, yellow, green and blue all seem pure colours, while orange and violet seem to be mixtures ; in the one case of red and yellow, in the other of red and blue. It is true that the red passes gradually into the yellow with changes in the relative proportions of the two components, and similarly the blue passes gradually into the red. At the same time red, yellow, blue, and probably green, are all experienced as pure, and without the trace of admixture of another or other colours.

When the physicist, from his own physical standpoint, proceeds to study the phenomena of colour-vision, and particularly of colour-blindness, he naturally starts from the spectrum. The more consistently he adheres to his physical standpoint, the greater the certainty that he will take a biased and incomplete view of the facts. If he holds fast to his spectrum basis, he is almost bound to force psychological and physiological facts into a physical mould, and to lop off or distort such as do not conform to the mould. Moreover, he will almost certainly place the emphasis wrongly, and he is also more than likely to employ a technique and methods of investigation, which are patently defective to the psychologist or physiologist.

It is obvious then that theories of colour-vision must start from the psychological facts, and must be, in the first instance, psychological, whatever the physicist may have to say later regarding them. It is from this point of view that the phenomena of colour-blindness must be approached. The scientific importance of colour-blindness depends on its significance with reference to theories of colour-vision. Hence the fundamental importance of a precise knowledge of the psychological phenomena of colour-blindness. The value of the work done by Dr Collins consists in the fact that she has shown with great clearness by her investigations the real nature of the psychological phenomena. Other investigators have had more cases of colour-blindness under observation—some have had many more—but, so far as I am aware, no other investigator has been so entirely free from prejudice in seeking to get at the facts of the colour experience of the colour-blind. As we have seen, this ought to have been the first point determined, but preoccupation with some colour theory or other has generally been an obstacle, and colour theories have suffered accordingly.

There is still more to be said for the kind of investigation carried out by Dr Collins. Not only are the facts she studies of the first importance from the point of view of colour vision theories ; they are also of great general interest. To be blind to the colour of objects and yet see the objects with perfect distinctness appears so strange and paradoxical that the ordinary man can hardly fail to be interested in knowing the kind of experience the colour-blind person has. This is exactly the same kind of knowledge as the psychologist seeks. It is also exactly the kind of knowledge that the investigations of Dr Collins yield, and it is the kind of knowledge, as we have just seen, that supplies the essential basis for a valid theory of colour-vision.

A considerable proportion of the most recent work on colour-blindness has been done by physicists, and much of it suffers from the defects incident to their method of approach. The best recent work, however, is that done by Edridge-Green. Among modern students of colour-blindness no one has had so wide an experience of the phenomena, and no one has done more to devise means for protecting the community against the dangers involved in colour-blindness in connection with certain important occupations. Dr Collins has much to say regarding the work done by Edridge-Green. Unfortunately, Edridge-Green, too, has come to his facts with a theory, and has to some extent forced his facts to fit the theory. On the one hand, he begins with the spectrum, and bases his whole interpretation of his facts upon that. On the other hand, he formulates a hypothesis to explain how the colour sense of the human being developed in the course of racial history, and again, to some extent, fits his facts to his hypothesis. The bearing of the facts, ascertained by Dr Collins on this theory and hypothesis, is, perhaps, worthy of passing notice.

Taking an evolutionary view, Edridge-Green supposes that for primitive vision the spectrum was uncoloured, but showed differences of brightness only. That is to say, it was seen as a band of varying shades of grey, and thus it is seen by the totally colour-blind, who represent this primitive stage. The first stage in the development of colour-vision was marked by the ability to distinguish the two extremes of the spectrum—the red and the violet ends respectively—the middle portion being still seen as grey, or being, as far as colour is concerned, a neutral band. Further development consisted in the filling-in of the neutral band with colours.

All this is pure speculation, and Dr Collins has apparently proved that in the main it is not supported by the facts. The first stage in the development of colour-vision ought to be represented by an extreme case of dichromatism—or red-green blindness—like the case of " J " recorded by Dr Collins. For " J," however, both the red and the violet ends of the spectrum were colourless. It is true he has a broad neutral band in the middle of the spectrum. But we must also note that he has another, and complementary, broad neutral band from red, through the purples and violets, to blue. This whole area is for him black or dark grey. It is not at all clear why, on an evolutionary view, one must assume that the extremes of the spectrum are first distinguished. Why not the maximal differences in brightness, that is, the yellow and the violet-blue? According to the findings of Dr Collins, this last represents more or less the condition of " J's " colour-vision. But Edridge-Green would apparently argue that cases like " J " really see violets and reds ; only they call reds yellow, and violets blue. The conclusive answer is that " J," at any rate, does nothing of the sort. He sees neither reds nor violets.

This matter of the double " neutral band " is of special interest and importance. By a " neutral band " is meant a band of what is to the normal eye colour, which is to the colour-blind eye colourless or grey. To illustrate the actual phenomena, let me take a case not studied by Dr Collins. A student, who had heard that we were investigating colour-blindness in the laboratory, came up one day and offered himself as a subject. He knew that he was colour-blind—slightly, he thought, but as a matter of fact he was markedly and typically red-green blind. In one test with our Bradley Paper Test, I handed the subject a dark olive-green card, and asked him to match the card on the sheets of colours. He matched it among the greens, fairly accurately—it was either of two, he said, and one was correct. Then I asked him, pointing to the extreme reds and purples, if he could match it there. Again he found a match. Lastly, I called his attention to the greys, and for a third time he found a match. A dark olive-green, a dark purple-red, and a dark grey were apparently all for him the same colour.

Dr Collins got confirmatory results with various subjects and various tests. That for partial colour-blinds, then, of the red-green type, there exists a colourless or grey band in the green region of the spectrum, admits of no doubt. That this band is of varying breadth in different subjects, as Edridge-Green contends, is also definitely established by Dr Collins. But, if our investigations are based on the spectrum, and we are not dealing with extreme cases like " J," we can have no suspicion of a complementary neutral band beyond the red of the spectrum. Thus we entirely miss a fact of the greatest significance for any theory of colour-vision. Apparently this is a fact which Edridge-Green has missed. Perhaps nothing could throw into clearer relief the inade-

B

quacy of a study of colour-blindness based on the spectrum, or the dangers lying in wait for the theorist who fails to distinguish between physical colour and physiological or psychological colour.

If the Edridge-Green colour theory is untenable, it must be confessed that several other colour theories, especially those based on physical data, are not in any better case. Hardly any colour theory, in fact, comes through the ordeal scatheless. As we have just seen, Edridge-Green's contention that there is gradation of colour defect is entirely substantiated by the investigations of Dr Collins. This highly significant fact would seem to involve some modification of most existing colour theories. There is, indeed, considerable evidence, some of which we shall consider later, pointing to the conclusion that the conditions determining colour sensations are by no means so simple as the leading colour theories would seem to imply.

Another interesting fact established by Dr Collins, which would seem to be significant for a colour theory, is that the colour-blind individual possesses a definite colour system, and apparently the colour system of each individual has characteristics of its own, which it is very difficult to interpret as due merely to the extent of the defect. The fact that the partially colour-blind individual possesses a definite colour system is of considerable psychological interest. Dr Collins found that even where colours were wrongly named they were never named in haphazard fashion. Of course, the confusions characteristic of colour-blindness were present, owing to the existence of neutral bands in the colour circle, but apart from these—and even the confusions presented a certain regularity and consistency—there was every evidence of a definite colour system. The other point—that the colour system of each individual has characteristics of its own—is somewhat more doubtful. Differences of nomenclature would apparently account for a considerable portion of the evidence on which this conclusion is based.

Bearing somewhat closely upon this same point is the discussion by Dr Collins of the experiments which were devised to throw light upon colour experiences designated by colour names not employed by the normal individual, such as "greenish-red" and "reddish-green." For normal colour-vision these terms can have no meaning. They are employed, however, with moderate frequency by colour-blinds. Several previous investigators have placed the fact on record, and Dr Collins found these or similar terms employed by half her subjects. As we have just seen, colour-blinds do not name colours in haphazard fashion. Hence it becomes an interesting problem to determine precisely what they mean by "reddish-green" or "greenish-red," and why they use such terms. The solution Dr Collins offers is at least plausible. She suggests that, though the individuals in question are blind to red for practical purposes, it is nevertheless exerting an influence on their colour experience. Thus their "reddish-green" may be a colour which the normal individual does not experience at all. In any case, the name is apparently always given to a colour that borders on one of the neutral zones. One might at first think that there was a simple solution. If the neutral zone which is seen as grey is called green, then at its margin towards the red end of the spectrum might we not expect to get a colour called "reddish green"? There are two difficulties. In the first place, ought we not rather to get "yellowish-green"? In the second place, there are two neutral zones, as we have already seen. In the one neutral zone the grey is bordered on the left by the yellows, on the right by the blues ; in the other neutral zone the grey is bordered on the left by the blues, on the right by the yellows. Dr Collins finds that there are undoubtedly two regions of the colour circle termed " reddish-green." Both are to the left of the yellow and the right of the blue. One is in the orange-yellow region, the other in the purple. This certainly suggests a sensitivity to red. It should, however, be noted that there may be a third region, in the other neutral zone, to which the term is applied, which would give rise to difficulties the solution of which is not at present apparent.

It must be remembered that Dr Collins finds much additional evidence for her view that some dichromates, though they do not see red as the normal individual sees it, and in certain circumstances confuse red with green, are nevertheless to some extent sensitive to red rays. It seems also that they may be more sensitive to red rays than to green rays. This is again theoretically important, if it should prove to be really the case. It involves somewhat formidable difficulties for one group of existing colour theories, namely, the group derived from or associated with the Hering four-colour theory. This is all the more interesting, because, on the whole, the findings of Dr Collins tend to support this type of theory.

Not only are the investigations of Dr Collins theoretically significant, but some of her practical results are also highly interesting and important. One of her main objects, as we have seen, was to institute a comparison of the various methods of testing for colour-blindness, in order to evaluate the different tests. She comes to the conclusion that the Edridge-Green lantern is for practical purposes the best test of all. But the employment of the Edridge-Green lantern requires that a considerable amount of time should be devoted to each individual case examined, and demands also something of the nature of laboratory facilities. It is, therefore, as it were, earmarked for use in all doubtful cases—a kind of final court of appeal. For a rapid preliminary examination, however, some other, and simpler, method of testing is desirable. Dr Collins finds that much simpler methods are reliable to a surprising extent, provided reasonable precautions are taken. The agreement in the conclusions reached on the basis of the different test methods is really astonishing. Stilling's Tables, Nagel's Cards, Holmgren's Wools, our own Bradley Colour Sheets, all give results in close agreement with one another, and with the results obtained with the Edridge-Green Lantern.

The rehabilitation of the old Holmgren Wool Test ought to be specially noted. There has long been well-nigh general agreement that this test is unreliable. This is more than a little curious in the light of the results obtained by Dr Collins. One cannot help wondering how many of those who so freely condemn the wool test have ever given it a fair trial. It is true that Dr Collins has her own method of administering the test, and particularly her own test skeins. She finds that the test skeins suggested by Holmgren do *not* give reliable results. But in view of her results it seems clear that, if the test skeins are selected on the basis of the knowledge we now possess of colour-blindness, few, if any, "dangerous" colour-blinds would escape even the despised wool test. Of course, the test skeins cannot be chosen at random ; the whole test depends on their careful selection. It is also interesting to see that, in this and other tests, Dr Collins finds that the naming by the subjects of the colours used is itself a method of testing for colour defect that frequently throws valuable additional light on the nature of the defect.   In this she is once more in agreement with Edridge-Green.

Perhaps something ought to be said regarding the limits to which Dr Collins has thought fit to confine her work. The title "Colour-Blindness" suggests a treatment of all varieties of colour-blindness.   Is the reader to understand that all varieties are represented by the cases studied and described by Dr Collins?   The answer is in the negative. She has herself indicated as much in the opening chapter. Colour-blindness may be either congenital or acquired. All the cases described are cases of congenital colour-blindness.   It may be either partial or total.   Again, all the cases described are cases of partial colour-blindness, though graded and extending nearly to the extreme state of total.   Partial colour-blindness may be either red-green or blue-yellow.   All the cases described are cases of red-green colour-blindness.   Finally, there may apparently be two varieties of all types of colour-blindness —a variety with normal length of spectrum, and a variety with shortened spectrum.   The exact significance of these two varieties is by no means clear, but both varieties of the red-green blind are represented in the cases described.

The reason for restricting detailed description to the varieties of red-green colour-blindness was simply that the cases observed and studied all belonged to this category.   The work of Dr Collins is intended to represent in the main her own observations and results.   In this lies its chief value.   She notices briefly the other types of colour-blindness that have been recorded.   But there was no object to be served in giving at second-hand a detailed description of these types.   The brief notice given, together with the appended bibliography, will enable any reader who so desires to go to the original records of these other types.   The present work, therefore, is not meant to be a compilation from such records, but itself an account at first-hand of actual observations. From the time when Dalton (1766–1844) made a study of his own case many records of colour-blind cases have been made and published, both on the continent and in this country.   Hence it may be asked further whether it was necessary to add to these records, and why.   The answer is that it was necessary, because of the fact that, in spite of the numerous records of cases of colour-blindness, there is still much uncertainty regarding the psychological phenomena.   So far as Dr Collins has contributed to the removal of this uncertainty her records were well worth making and publishing.

Writers treating of the practical bearing of colour-blindness are apt to confine their attention to the case of the railwayman and the sailor.   Even thus they find no difficulty in showing its great practical significance. But its practical bearings are much wider.   Dr Collins, in her closing chapter, has enumerated the chief occupations in which colour-blindness is a serious handicap. The general plan of her work afforded no opportunity of developing and illustrating this particular aspect.   A single illustration, therefore, might be given here, in order to assist the reader in visioning her results from a practical angle.   The illustration is selected from George Combe's *System of Phrenology*.   In a book issuing from the George Combe Department of Psychology it is fitting that there should be some allusion to his treatment of the subject, all the more when this treatment is among the earliest appearing in any psychological textbook— Combe's *System of Phrenology* may be so described.

In discussing the organ of " Colouring "—located by the phrenologists of the time in the middle of the eyebrow—

Combe begins by criticizing Dugald Stewart's expression
of opinion that inability to name colours is generally due
to defects in conception rather than in perception.[1] Had
he read further in the passage he quotes, he would have
seen that Dugald Stewart admits that colour-blindness
does exist in certain cases, though he implies that these
are rare. Combe, however, goes on to cite some cases
of colour-blindness, at least one of which—Milne—is a
very typical case. Milne " was bound apprentice to a
draper, and continued in his service for three years and
a half. During two years he fell into considerable mistakes
about colours, but this was attributed to inexperience,
and ignorance of the names of the tints. At length,
however, when he was selling a piece of olive-green
corduroy for breeches, the purchaser requested strings
to tie them with ; and Mr Milne was proceeding to cut
off what he considered the best match, when the person
stopped him, and requested strings of the same colour
as the cloth. Mr Milne begged him to point out a colour
to please himself ; and he selected, of course, a green
string. When he was gone Mr Milne was so confident
that he himself was right, and the purchaser wrong, that
he cut off a piece of the string which he intended to give,
and a piece of that which had been selected, and carried
both home, with a piece of the cloth also, and
showed them to his mother. She then told him
that *his ribbon* was a *bright scarlet*, and *the other* a
grass-green."[2]

Milne's condition is clearly indicated by Combe's
further description of the case. " As to the different
colours, he knows blues and yellows certainly ; but he
cannot distinguish browns, greens and reds. A brown and

[1] *Elements of the Philosophy of the Human Mind*, Chapter 3.
[2] *System of Phrenology*. Vol. II, p. 57 (5th ed., 1853). Italics are
his.

green he cannot discriminate or name when apart ; but when together he sees a difference between them. Blue and pink, when about the same shade, and seen in daylight, appear to him to be of the colour of the sky, which he calls blue ; but seen in candle-light, the pink appears like a dirty buff, and the blue retains the appearance which it had in daylight. The grass appears to him more like an orange than any other coloured object with which he is acquainted. Indigo, violet, and purple appear only different shades of one colour, darker or lighter, but not differing in their bases."[1]

All this is very typical, and the reader will find that practically every one of Dr Collins' subjects presents similar phenomena. Her fuller analysis, however, brings out the differences as well as the resemblances in colour-blind cases. While these differences are of considerable general interest and of great theoretical importance, the points in which all resemble one another are probably of greater practical significance. One and all, if placed in a situation analogous to that in which Milne was placed in the draper's shop, would have the same kinds of difficulties to face.

Of course, if colour-blindness were a rarely occurring condition, the fact that it constituted a serious handicap in various occupations would be of relatively small significance. But it is by no means rare. It is true that total colour-blindness is very rarely met with, and blue-yellow colour-blindness occurs so seldom that there is still considerable doubt whether it exists as a congenital condition. But red-green colour-blindness is in an entirely different category. Among men its frequency of occurrence is about one in every twenty or thirty ; among women it occurs much less frequently—perhaps

[1] *Loc. cit.*

about one in every thousand.[1] A condition that occurs
among men so frequently as this, and that involves, to
such an extent, incapacity for the performance of various
duties and various kinds of work, clearly demands the
most serious consideration, in order that danger to the
community or hardship to the individual may be avoided
or minimized. The matter is sufficiently important to
justify the testing of all children during the school period,
and in connection with the ordinary medical examination.
Much individual hardship might be avoided in this way ;
the precautions against danger to the community are
already comparatively sufficient and satisfactory.

The herditary character of colour-blindness was early
recognized. The actual facts, however, appear to be
somewhat complex. We have come across several cases
where brother and sister both showed colour-weakness,
but on being tested the brother was found to be definitely
colour-blind, while the sister could only be characterized
as colour-weak. It is known also that colour-blindness
may occur in males of one generation, be latent in the
next generation, especially in a female generation, and
occur once more in males of the succeeding generation.
It has been said that its inheritance passes by the female
line. Whether the data available are sufficient to establish
this or not, it is certain that the colour-blindness is for
the most part latent in the female, though possibly indicating its latency by colour-weakness.

It is an interesting psychological exercise for the normal
individual to try to construct in imagination the world
as it must appear to the colour-blind. In the case of the
totally colour-blind, such an imaginative construction
would eliminate from the world as the normal individual
sees it all colour, and everything the apprehension or

---

[1] *See* below, p. 220.

appreciation of which depends on colour. The world
would become a world of black, white, and various shades
of grey—a world of light and shade only, like a landscape
in black and white. The blue of the sky and the sea,
the green of the field and the purple of the heather, the
bright hues of flowers, all these would have no place in
the totally colour-blind's experience of the world around
him. So, too, with respect to the people in his world.
The changing seasons are marked for the normal individual
by nothing so much as the changing hues of the landscape.
These changing hues would not exist for the colour-blind
save as changes in light and shade. Apart from changes
in detail, such as those caused by the leaves coming on the
trees, there would be little difference between winter
and summer.

For the partially colour-blind the world of Nature and
man does not wear quite so sombre an aspect. The red-
green blind sees blues and yellows. Hence a yellowish-
red or a yellowish-green will be seen as yellow. Thus
for Milne grass appeared the same colour as an orange—
presumably yellow. Purples will be blue, if there is
sufficient blue in them to be apprehended. The wealth
of colour in the world of Nature and man will therefore
be greatly diminished, though the result will not be quite
so drab a universe as for the totally colour-blind. The
results obtained by Dr Collins enable us to form a fairly
accurate idea of the colours in this world. If there is a
partial blue-yellow colour-blindness, the visible world of
an individual so affected must be exceedingly bizarre
measured according to normal standards, characterized
as it would be by greens and reds alone.

One of the tests employed by Dr Collins throws some
light on the emotional life of colour-blind individuals so
far as that depends on colours. This is the investigation

of colour preference. Colour preference depends partly on associations. It depends also on the direct effects of colours. In either case we should expect that colour-blindness would exert a marked influence on the individual's affective reactions to colours. That it does so appears at once from the results of the colour preference experiments given by Dr Collins.

There can be no doubt that congenital colour-blindness, either red-green or total, represents in some sort a reversion to a more primitive stage of development, as far as the organ of vision is concerned. Where precisely this stage is normally found in the history of the race is a more difficult question. Lord Avebury thought he had satisfactory evidence of colour discrimination among bees and wasps, but subsequent investigators have not confirmed his conclusions, and in general have found that his results can be otherwise explained. Investigations in animal psychology by Hess and others would, however, seem to prove conclusively that colours are discriminated as far down the animal scale as the birds. On the other hand, arguing on the basis of language, various writers have come to the conclusion that the colour sense in the human being is of comparatively late development.

The language evidence depends on the presence or absence of colour words in a language. Thus, if there is no word in a language for green or blue or yellow, it is argued that the people or tribe in question are insensitive to green or blue or yellow, as the case may be. If we argue on this basis we must come to the conclusion that the Greeks of the Homeric period were insensitive to blue, since they used the same word to designate the blue of the sky, as they used of any dark grey object. And generally we find a word for red before we find a word for blue. But evidence of this sort is obviously inconsistent with evidence obtained from other and more reliable sources. Actual investigation of the colour sense of primitive peoples has led to the conclusion that there is no evidence to be obtained for the view that their colour sense is radically different from that of modern highly civilized peoples. Exploration of the field of colour in the retina shows also that the marginal and least highly developed zone is colour-blind, the most highly developed central zone is sensitive to all colours, and the zone intermediate in position and in development is red-green blind.

Wundt has shown the fallacy of the philological argument in conclusive fashion.[1] He points out that the aim of language is the expression of thought, and intercommunication, not scientific analysis. Names for colours come into use only when they are required for practical purposes, and the scope of the practical extends as civilized life develops in complexity. Hence the earliest colour names are names of objects which have immediate practical importance or excite strong feelings, and have also a distinctive colour. Language, therefore, can supply little or no evidence regarding the development of the colour sense. One might ask, how does this bear upon colour-naming tests? Obviously in the naming tests employed by Dr Collins the evidence from language is of an entirely different type, though even in this case we must be careful in the use of our data, and must check with data obtained in other and purely objective ways.

There is one further point to which reference might be made in conclusion. In our ordinary everyday way of thinking we regard white, black and grey as colours equally with blue, yellow, green and red. The theory of colour vision associated with the name of Hering is in

---

[1] *Lectures on Human and Animal Psychology* (Trans. by Creighton and Titchener) p. 101, *seq.*

part founded upon this ordinary view. To the two antagonistic processes underlying our sensory experience of blue and yellow, green and red, respectively, a third, underlying our experience of black and white, is added. But careful consideration of the facts obtained by Dr Collins, as well as of other facts of vision, makes it clear that black and white, with the intermediate greys, are in a different category from the spectral colours. The mere fact that blindness to black and white would be, not colour-blindness, but actual blindness—absence of vision—is itself conclusive. An individual who cannot see reds and greens, or blues and yellows, can still see the objects so coloured to the normal eye ; an individual who cannot see black, white or grey cannot see objects.

The fact seems to be that in vision we have two separate sense departments, and at least two separate " end-organs." Seeing and seeing colours are two distinct types of sensory experience. If this is so, then red and green on the one hand, and white and black on the other, are both in a sense antagonistic, but antagonistic in different ways. If we mix on a colour mixer a red disc with a disc of its complementary green, beginning with the red pure, and gradually adding more and more of the green, we get first of all a gradual diminution in the saturation of the red with no change of hue, then a grey and finally a green with increasing saturation, but no change of hue, till we come to the full green. What has apparently happened in the course of the experiment is that the added green has neutralized more and more of the red until it is all neutralized, and then a less and less proportion of the green has been neutralized by the red. But the red and green discs have affected the end-organ for light and shade also, so that when both colours are neutralized this effect only is left, and we get the sensation of grey. On the other hand, if we mix a white disc and a black disc in the same way, we get a characteristically different result. We do not get a change from a diminishing saturation of white to an increasing saturation of black, through a grey, but a continuous series of greys, of which the white and the black are merely the two extremes.

This experiment enables us to understand the condition of the eye in colour-blindness, as also the nature of the colour-blind individual's experience of colours. The colour-blindness must be due to the absence or inactivity of some kind of " end-organ," which can be absent or inactive without light and shade vision being affected. Hence the colours which the colour-blind subject does not see as colours are nevertheless seen as greys. If, with a red-green colour-blind subject we perform the experiment with the red and green discs, we find that grey is seen from start to finish. It merely changes in shade. Hence the red-green colour-blind will match, as Dr Collins has found and described, greens, browns, and reds with one another and with grey, simply because they are all greys for him. Keeping these facts in view, we shall more readily comprehend some of the apparently extraordinary results which Dr Collins has obtained.

J. DREVER.

George Combe Department of Psychology,
University of Edinburgh.

COLOUR-BLINDNESS

CHAPTER I

INTRODUCTORY

THE study of colour-blindness has been somewhat retarded
by the concomitant study of colour theories. The
majority of investigators have started out unduly biased
by their favourite theory and have examined colour-
blinds from this prejudiced standpoint. The result is
that a great deal of unnecessary confusion has gathered
round this subject, which has ultimately caused an obscur-
ing of the real issues. Attempts have been made from
time to time to get away from theories, but, on the whole,
these have proved futile, and the results achieved are
only gradually permeating the literature of the subject.
Yet even in the highest authoritative references to colour-
blindness, it is amazing to find that a description of the
defect is inevitably given along the lines of some particular
theory, although it must be admitted that some authors
take the precaution of inserting a note to the effect that
such a description holds only if that theory be accepted.

Dr Hayes, who revolts against this method, states that
" the general topic of colour-blindness is still in a
state which many psychologists consider to be most
disgraceful to their science. One reason for this backward
condition is undoubtedly to be found in the extreme
complexity of the subject, and the enormous variations

from case to case ; but an even greater obstacle to the progress of knowledge has been the almost universal practice of studying and classifying cases under the domination of some preconceived colour-theory."[1]

The division of partial colour-blinds into Red-blind, Green-blind, and Violet-blind, following the Young-Helmholtz theory, is the most noted example of this falsifying of results. It is a more or less established fact that the so-called red-blind is also blind to green, and the so-called green-blind, blind to red, yet this terminology is still frequently applied to describe this colour anomaly. And what is more surprising is that in detailing tests useful in examining colour-blinds the tests are vitiated by the theory lying behind them. The Holmgren wool test, a splendid one for dichromates, is still seemingly employed to select out the red-blinds from the green-blinds, and Holmgren's coloured plate showing the matches which the two types of colour-blinds make is often referred to as authoritative. We still find, in so recent a book as Abney's *Researches in Colour Vision*, instructions similar to Holmgren's own. " If in the second test, he selects with purple only green and grey, or one of them, he is completely green-blind. The red-blind never selects the colours taken by the green-blind, and *vice versa*."[2] This division of the colour-blinds into groups, which are totally at variance with the known facts, has done much to spread false ideas of the defect, and progress has been considerably impeded. The wool test, as we shall see later, is excellent for diagnosis if we leave aside the implications on which it was based and reject the idea of a rigid classification.

---

[1] " The Colour Sensations of the Partially Colour-Blind," *American Journal of Psychology*, 1911, Vol. XXII, p. 369.
[2] Holmgren's own words. Quoted from a Translation by Jeffries in *Colour-Blindness : its Dangers and Detection*, p. 213.

The Helmholtz theory has been merely cited as an illustration of a theory predominating facts. There is no intention to decry the theory as an explanation of the various phenomena of colour defect. It has been modified since Young and Helmholtz first formulated it. But what must be emphasized is that its influence is clearly visible in the reports of many of the cases of dichromasy which have been investigated.

Brief Historical Survey

It is interesting to trace the illumination which has been gradually thrown upon this curious defect. As the experiments which are to be described later deal only with colour-blindness in its most common form, namely, blindness to red and green, only a brief account will be given of blue-yellow blindness and of total colour-blindness.

1. Red-Green Colour-Blindness

The earliest case on record seems to be that of Harris, the shoemaker, reported in 1777 by Mr Huddart in a letter to the Rev. J. Priestley. Mr Huddart writes " The account he (Harris) gave was this : that he had reason to believe other persons saw something in objects which he could not see ; that their language seemed to mark qualities with confidence and precision which he could only guess at with hesitation, and frequently with error. His first suspicion of this arose when he was about four years old. Having by accident found in the street a child's stocking, he carried it to a neighbouring house to inquire for the owner. He observed the people called it a *red* stocking, though he did not understand why they gave it that denomination, as he himself thought it completely described by being called a stocking." This seemed to imply a blindness to red, although Abney explains the defect as being one of green-blindness. " He observed also, that when young, other children could discern cherries on a tree by some pretended difference of colour, though he could only distinguish them from the leaves by their difference of size and shape. He observed, also, that by means of this difference of colour, they could see the cherries at a greater distance than he could, though he could see other objects at as great a distance as they ; that is, where the sight was not assisted by the colour." This seems to be the first scientific account of any abnormality in colour vision, although it must always have been a fairly common defect ; evidently it had existed undetected. This first account appears to be a description of a case of confusion of both red and green. It is interesting to note that Harris had two brothers who were similarly affected.

In 1794 Dalton's. description of his own case appeared[1] and attracted considerable attention—so much so that Daltonism became for long the name by which colour-blindness was described. He first became acquainted with his defect by observing a pink geranium in candle-light. " The flower was pink, but it appeared to me almost an exact sky-blue by day. In candle-light, however, it was astonishingly changed, not having then any blue in it, but being what I called *red*—a colour which forms a striking contrast to blue." He found on examination that his brother suffered from the same defect—showing, as in the case of Harris, the hereditary nature of the phenomenon. He further states that while he found that most people could distinguish six colours in the solar spectrum, his colour sensations were reduced to two, blue and yellow, or at the most three—blue, yellow,

[1] *Literary and Philosophical Society of Manchester.*

and purple. " My yellow comprehends the red, orange, yellow, and green of others ; and my blue and purple coincide with theirs. That part of the image which others call red appears to me little more than a shade, or defect of light ; after that, the orange, yellow, and green seem one colour, which descends pretty uniformly from an intense to a rare yellow, making what I should call different shades of yellow. The difference between the green part and the blue part is very striking to my eye; they seem to be strongly contrasted. That between the blue and purple is much less so. The purple appears to be blue, much darkened and condensed." This is an excellent description of a colour-blind. Dalton's defect was said to be due to an inability to see the colour red, and Daltonism accordingly sometimes stands for this particular form of colour-blindness. Dalton attributed his defect to the fact that one of the humours of his eye, probably the vitreous humour, was a colour medium, probably some modification of blue. But an examination of his eye after death did not support any such theory.

Goethe in 1812 in his *Theory of Colours*[1] described this defect of colour-blindness in the following manner. " We will here advert to a very remarkable state in which the vision of many persons is found to be. As it presents a deviation from the ordinary mode of seeing colours, it may be classed under morbid impressions ; but as it is consistent with itself, as it often occurs, may extend to several members of a family, and probably does not admit of cure, we may consider it as bordering only on the nosological cases." The two cases which Goethe was acquainted with saw white, grey, and black in the usual manner. They also saw yellow, red-yellow, and yellow-red, but they confused blue with pink, green with dark

[1] Translation by Eastlake.

orange, green and brown. " These persons saw fewer colours than other people, hence the confusion of different colours."

The next cases reported are in 1816–7 by Dr Nichols—one of a boy aged eleven, the other of a man aged forty-nine. They are both reported as making the typical mistakes of the red-green colour-blind. " The colour I am most at a loss with is green ; and in attempting to distinguish it from red, it is nearly guess-work. The different shades of red and green, I know not to which they belong ; but, when they are before me, I see a difference in the shade. Though I see different shades in looking at a rainbow, I should say it was a mixture of yellow and blue—yellow in the centre and blue towards the edge."

In 1837 Seebeck gave a detailed analysis of the several cases which he had investigated. He found he could divide his subjects into two classes based on the difference in the length of the spectrum which was visible to them. This led later to the classification of deuteranopes whose colour system is reduced to blue and yellow, but who have a normal length of spectrum, and protanopes who likewise see blue and yellow but whose spectrum is shortened at the red end. This is the most marked differentiation of the present day and has been generally accepted.

Sir John Herschel, however, was the first to put forward the dichromic explanation of colour-blindness. He pointed out in his well-known article on " Light," written for the *Encyclopædia Metropolitana*,[1] that certain individuals could only distinguish two colours, blue and yellow. This seems to have been the first positive statement of the diagnosis of the defect—the former cases reported being merely descriptive. Herschel considered Dalton's

[1] 1845, § 507.

case as coming under this category, but this explanation was objected to by Prof. George Wilson. Wilson had taken particular interest in Dalton's case, and considered that Dalton did not show signs of blindness to red.

In Wilson's book, *Researches on Colour-Blindness* (published in 1855), he describes a large number of cases which he had personally studied. He discusses the various theories which had been formulated at that time and examines many of the phenomena which had been observed to accompany the defect. He points out, for example, that some Daltonians, as he calls them, can distinguish colours by other means than vision, " Slight differences in shape, accidental rough points, folds, wrinkles, and the like " and touch. " Wools dyed with certain compounds are much harsher to the touch than those dyed with others ; the mineral pigments, such as Prussian blue, or chromate of lead, in general producing rougher surfaces than the organic dyes, such as indigo. A wool dyed with a mineral might thus be distinguished by the touch, from one dyed with a vegetable red, although the colour-blind eye could detect no difference between their tints."[1] An important step was taken by Wilson in testing the colour-blinds. He used a large number of samples of coloured wool, coloured paper and glasses, which the examinee arranged in groups—this is the method so splendidly adapted later by Holmgren in his investigations.

Clerk Maxwell in the same year, in a communication to the Royal Society of Edinburgh, on " Experiments on Colour as Perceived by the Eye, with Remarks on Colour-Blindness," seemed to agree with Prof. Wilson in regarding dichromic cases of colour-blindness as not firmly established. " In experiments made with the pure spectrum,

[1] p. 116.

it appears that, though the red appears much more obscure than the other colours, it is not invisible." He adopted a new method of experiment, by revolving colour discs and forming colour equations. The discs were slipped on a top or teetotum which consisted of a flat disc of tin plate and a vertical axis of ivory. The axis passed through the centre of the disc, and the quantity of each colour exposed could be measured by a graduation on the rim of the disc, which was divided into one hundred parts. " The principal use of the top is to obtain colour equations. These are got by producing, by two different combinations of colours, the same mixed tint. For this purpose there is another set of discs, half the diameter of the others, which lie above them, and by which the second combination of colours is formed."[1] Prof. Clerk Maxwell was an adherent of the theory first postulated by Thos. Young in 1801, and later adopted by Helmholtz.[2] This theory, postulated to explain the general facts of colour vision, assumed there were three elementary colours corresponding to which there were three nerve fibres in the retina. The stimulation of the first aroused the sensation of red, of the second green, and of the third violet. In other words, the action of the long wave end of the spectrum affected the first, of the middle wave length, the second, and of the short wave end, the third, but light of all kinds excited all three fibres though in varying degrees. In the modern exposition of the theory the nerve fibres have been replaced by three photochemical substances. Young's theory received scant attention until it was revived by Helmholtz, and later upheld by Clerk Maxwell. It was easy to assume in the case of colour-blindness the simple explanation that absence of one of the fibres was sufficient

[1] Quoted from a letter written by Clerk Maxwell to Dr G. Wilson, 1855.
[2] *Vide infra*, p. 31.

to cause the defect. The absence of the red element caused an inability to see reds, lack of the green element a corresponding inability to see greens, and possibly a third case existed in which the lack of the third element gave rise to violet blindness. For a time the facts of colour-blindness seemed strongly in favour of this classification. Colour-blinds were either red-blind, green-blind, or violet-blind. The red-blind were blind to red, but could see the remaining two colours, green and violet ; the green-blind were blind to green, but could see red and violet. Maxwell's colour equations seemed to be consistent with this explanation.

At an early stage, however, doubts began to arise, and in an account by Dr Pole of his own case (he was a red-green colour-blind)[1] we find that he vigorously protests against the prevailing beliefs, and gives a careful analysis of his own colour vision as evidence. He had been pronounced red-blind by Maxwell, and green-blind by Holmgren, who based his conclusions on his wool test. Dr Pole repudiated both suggestions and claimed that the true solution was that he was blind to both colours. He based his evidence on a large array of facts.[2] First, the testimony of the colour-blind themselves, who, whether they were acclaimed as red-blind or green-blind, unanimously asserted that their colour sensations were confined to blue and yellow.

Secondly, the study of acquired colour-blindness.

Thirdly, colour-blindness of one eye only.

Von Hippel's case, reported in 1880, attracted considerable attention. The subject, a young man who knew nothing of his defect, and who came to von Hippel for spectacles to cure double vision, was found to be

[1] *Proceedings of Royal Society of London*, 1856.
[2] *Transactions of the Royal Society of Edinburgh*, 1893.

colour-blind in one eye. His left eye was normal, his right was dichromic. His peripheral vision was tested and with the right eye he was found to confuse red and green with yellow. Further tests with Stilling's pseudo-isochromatic tables, Holmgren's wools, and von Hippel's photometer confirmed the result. The colour sensations which the subject experienced with his right eye were blue and yellow. Von Hippel diagnosed this case as one of red-green blindness—with spectrum of normal length.

Holmgren diagnosed the same case and proclaimed it to be one of red-blindness with shortened spectrum. In accord with the Helmholtz theory, as presented in the first edition of the *Physiological Optics*, 1867, the subject was able to see a greenish yellow and a blue tending to violet.

Von Hippel re-tested his subject and substantiated his claim that the spectrum was not shortened and that the colours seen by the colour-blind eye and verified by the normal eye were blue and yellow. This was the first case of monocular vision reported, verifying the dichromasy of colour-blindness.

Holmgren ultimately agreed that blue and yellow were the only colours seen, and von Kries, also a staunch supporter of the Young-Helmholtz theory, noted the result. They refused to admit, however, that such a case affected the validity of the theory, but agreed that the application of it to explain dichromatism was no longer tenable.

Fourthly, the analogy of peripheral colour-blindness.

The result was overwhelming evidence that the colour system of the colour-blind was composed of blue and yellow As Dr Pole so justly remarks, "Not a fact of any kind to lead to the belief that the sensation is not yellow, but red or green. Nothing but a peculiar inference drawn

empirically from a certain theory which, though command-
ing the greatest respect in regard to colour vision generally,
does not in the least necessitate the form of application
to colour-blindness under which this inference has been
drawn."[1]

We find Helmholtz in 1892 referring to the former
explanation as an "old attempt to explain colour-
blindness." He adopted blue and yellow as the two
fundamental sensations of the colour-blind, and declared
that the absence of one of the elements no longer explained
the defect. The three fundamental colours, red, green,
and violet, were changed as regards their degree of excitability. The sensation of yellow was said to arise from
the fact that the red and the green elements were equally
stimulated.

This solution was objected to by Hering[2] who had
postulated a different theory to explain the facts. His
theory of colour-vision assumed six simple visual sensations, white, black, yellow, blue, red, and green. These
can be arranged in pairs, white black, yellow blue, red
green, which are complementary to each other, and at
the same time antagonistic. The mixture of these six
colours in different proportions gives rise to all the colour
sensations.

From an examination of different cases, Hering concluded that the division into red and green blinds was a
false one—that the red-blind was also blind to green.
His explanation was, therefore, that the absence of the
red-green elements would meet the case, leaving blue and
yellow, black and white as the sensations of the colour-
blind. The spectrum would appear—in accordance with
the known facts—yellow and blue with different degrees

[1] Pole, *ibid.*
[2] *An Essay towards the Explanation of Colour-Blindness by the Theory
of Opposite Colours.*

of saturation. " The red-green blind patients always
point out pure yellow and blue correctly, and no two
colours in which blue, on the one hand, and yellow, on
the other, are prominent, are ever mistaken for each
other."[1]   Hering explained the two varieties of red-green
colour-blindness as due to differences in the macular
pigmentation.

Hering alluded to the new explanation of colour-
blindness offered by Helmholtz, namely, that the red and
green curves had become identical, and concluded " on
the whole, that if the Young-Helmholtz theory had not
been bequeathed to physiologists as a venerable legacy,
it would certainly never have been drawn from the
examination of the colour-blind."[2]

The results of these two great theories have been that
partial colour-blinds have been divided into classes—
three classes by the advocates of Helmholtz, red, green,
and violet—two classes by the advocates of Hering, red-
green blindness and blue-yellow blindness.

Von Kries suggested the terms deuteranopes and
protanopes to mark off the different types exclusive of
any particular theory. The deuteranopes are those
whose colour system is reduced to yellow and blue, but
who see colour throughout the whole length of the
spectrum ; the protanopes are those whose colour system
is reduced to yellow and blue, but whose spectrum is
shortened at the red end. In this second type the point
of maximum brightness has been found to be shifted
towards the green ; in other words, they show the Purkinje
phenomenon in ordinary light. Dr Rivers suggested the
two terms photerythrous and scoterythrous[3] to describe

[1] From a Translation by Pole, *Philosophical Magazine*, Vol. XXXVI,
1893.
[2] *Ibid.*, p. 194.
[3] " Vision," in Schäfer's *Text-book of Physiology*.

the two groups. He adopted the terms from Dr Verral, of Trinity College, Cambridge, but unfortunately they have not met with general acceptance.

The two, however, are not found sufficient to describe all cases which show deviation from the normal. Seebeck, even in 1837, found certain cases which he was reluctant to classify as colour-blinds, and yet they showed signs of abnormality. They seemed to be cases of weak colour vision. It was not until 1881, when Rayleigh reported the results of his experiments,[1] that these cases were understood. Rayleigh found that a number of individuals with otherwise normal vision were unequally sensitive to red and green. In equating red and green equal to yellow (since known as the Rayleigh equation) some were found to require far more red than the normal; others required an excess of green. Von Kries, in describing an extensive series of experiments, applied the name " anomalous trichromates " to them, and this term has gained universal currency. The anomalous trichromates see the three fundamental colours of Helmholtz in the spectrum but are unequally sensitive to red and green. Guttman advocated the terms "red-weak" and "green-weak," and distinguished seven characteristic symptoms which they manifested ; a reduced sensitivity to colour stimuli especially when the stimulus is of short duration, small area, and low intensity, a decidedly heightened colour contrast, difficulty in comparing colour tones of unequal brightness or saturation, and quick fatigue to colour stimuli. These seven inter-related symptoms form a complex state, so that the abnormality varies considerably with different individuals.

Nagel rejects the term colour-weakness as being too wide, and prefers the term anomalous trichromatism.

---

[1] *Nature*, 25, 64–6, 1881.

It is customary to divide these anomalous trichromates into two groups corresponding to the two groups of dichromatism—deuteranomalous trichromates whose sensitiveness to green is below normal and protanomalous trichromates whose sensitiveness to red is below normal.

Research on colour-blinds since has been carried out in the hope of solving various problems, or are merely descriptive. The followers of Helmholtz, such as Abney, have adopted new methods of studying the defect, all with a view of proving the favoured theory. It is interesting to note that Abney's luminosity test was adopted by the Board of Trade in 1912. The adherents of Hering have been equally assiduous in supporting their claims. New theories have arisen, each claiming to be a better interpretation of the facts, and a number of them have explained colour-blindness as a regression to a previous stage of colour evolution.

One large advance which has been made has been the devising of tests for practical use. It has long been recognized that red-green colour-blindness may be a danger to the community in such occupations where the distinction between red and green is of paramount importance, and accidents on sea and rail have often been attributed, and in some cases traced, to this cause.

One of the largest contributors of tests devised to pick out dangerous colour-blinds has been Professor Edridge-Green. In his capacity of Examiner to the Board of Trade, he has examined a large number of candidates, and has embodied his results in numerous publications. He rejects the simple classification of colour-blinds into dichromates, for he finds many grades and varieties of severity of the defect. The individual of normal vision can see six colours in the spectrum (sometimes seven), and he accordingly is ranked as a six-unit (or a seven-unit).

According to the number of colours he can perceive, an individual is a five, four, three, two, or a one-unit. The two extreme ends of the spectrum are the first to be seen red and violet—the dichromate therefore can see red and violet. But Edridge-Green points out that, as the colour perception improves, the red and violet will invade the grey and approach each other. When the whole of the grey has disappeared, the colours seen will not be red and violet, but blue and yellow. Yellow is the *centre* colour of the red unit and blue the *centre* colour of the violet unit. The three-unit sees red and violet, and a third colour, green, makes its appearance. The four-unit can see red, yellow, green, and violet, the five-unit red, yellow, green, blue, and violet, and the normal six-unit red, orange, yellow, green, blue, and violet. In addition to these classes, there are others distinguished by shortening either of the red or the violet end of the spectrum. The two-unit corresponds to the dichromate ; the three, four, and five-units are anomalous trichromates. This theory is interesting in showing the grading of the colour sense from the six or seven normal unit to the two, one, or none-unit class, which represents total colour-blindness.

Edridge-Green bases his results, published in *Colour-Blindness and Colour Perception*, on an examination of a hundred and sixteen cases. He has devised a pocket wool test ; a classification test ; a colour perception Spectro-meter, and constructed a lantern specially devised to detect dangerous colour-blinds. He rejects Holmgren's wool test as unsatisfactory, and attaches great importance to the colour names which the colour-blind employ. The dangerous colour-blinds, according to Edridge-Green, are :

1. Those who see three or less colours in the spectrum.

2. Those who, whilst being able to perceive a greater number of colours than three, have the red end of the spectrum shortened to a degree incompatible with their recognition of a red light at a distance of two miles.

3. Those who are unable to distinguish between the red, green, and white lights at the normal distance through defect or insensitiveness of the cerebro-retinal apparatus when the image on the retina is diminished in size[1] (*i.e.*, those of central scotoma).

Collins, who, in 1918,[2] carried out an examination of a thousand persons with the Edridge-Green lantern, confirms these results and marks as dangerously colour-blind the three classes enumerated above. His final judgment is, that the dangerous colour-blinds can be satisfactorily discovered by means of the Edridge-Green lantern.

Professor Hayes, in the *American Journal of Psychology*, 1911, gives the results of a series of experiments which he carried out with the intention of showing that dichromatism should be regarded as a limiting case. He asserts that there are mild cases of colour-blindness who can see red or green under favourable conditions, that there are protanopes who can see some greens, and deuteranopes who can see some reds. His main results are based on a case of monocular protanopia, and he gives convincing evidence that his subject in certain experiments could distinguish green. " If we grant that von Hippel's patient saw only blue and yellow, must we not also grant that Miss G. S. sees green, blue, and yellow? This assumption is supported by abundant indications that many of our

---

[1] *Hunterian Lectures on Colour-Vision and Colour-Blindness*, p. 47.
[2] *Public Health Bulletin*, No. 92, Wash. Govt. Printing Office, 1918.

colour-blinds possess a similar sensation to red or to green."
In confirmation he adds, in a footnote, that Nagel reported
that, among thirty dichromates, both protanopes and
deuteranopes, examined by him, none failed to recognize
various shades of red when a sufficiently large area of the
retina was stimulated. Professor Hayes' ultimate conclusion is, that there is a large mass of evidence which
points out the presence of sensations of red or green in the
colour systems of the partially colour-blind. He asserts
that a strict classification of colour defectives is necessarily
artificial, and that there are numerous transitional cases
between normality and total colour-blindness. Dichromasy should be regarded as an extreme variation, and not
as a typical condition of the partially colour-blind.

2. *Blue-Yellow Blindness*

Congenital blue-yellow blindness has not been definitely
established, although one or two seemingly authentic cases
have been reported. It is generally considered to be patho-
logical in character and to accompany definite changes in the
retina. Parsons[1] points out that " it is simulated in cases
of jaundice and sclerosis of the crystalline lens, these being
due to absorption by yellow pigment." Abney[2] and Hess[3]
have found that the same defect may arise in cases where
the pigmentation of the macula is unusually dense.
Although the majority of cases are of this type, cases
have also been recorded in which the defect seems to be
congenital in nature. Such a case has been reported by
Richardson.[4]

Blue-yellow blindness, as may have been gathered from
the foregoing remarks, occurs very rarely. As a result its

---

[1] *An Introduction of Colour-Vision*, p. 181. (All references are to
1st Edition).
[2] *Proceedings of the Royal Society of London*, 1891, 49.
[3] Hess, *Arch. f. Anat.*, 61, 29, 1908.
[4] *Psychological Bulletin*, Vol. VIII, 1911, 55–6, 214–5; *American
Journal of Psychology*, Vol. XXXIV, 1923, 157–184.
D

existence has been disputed and its investigation has not been so thoroughly undertaken as in the case of the other form of partial colour-blindness. As its name implies, blue and yellow are the confusion colours, and as there is no danger arising from inability to distinguish red from green, this type of colour-blindness has not the same practical importance which might necessitate a closer analysis of its characteristics. It is, however, of considerable theoretical importance.

In a manner analogous to the type of colour-blindness considered in Section 1, this second form of partial colour-blindness has received various names according to the theory under which it has been discussed. If we regard it from the standpoint of the Young-Helmholtz theory, we find it described as *violet*-blindness, or as Maxwell prefers to call it—still in terms of the same theory—*blue*-blindness. It is caused by the absence of the third colour-perceiving element. This leaves the other two colour elements, red and green, as clear colours for such abnormals. Theoretically the spectrum of the violet-blind must be represented as follows : " The *red* is a purer red colour (not yellowish) than normal red, but still less ' saturated.' The more it inclines towards orange, the more strongly luminous it is, but is at the same time less ' saturated,' more whitish. The *yellow* is, as it were, a combination of almost equal proportions of the fundamental colours that form white. *Green* is a strongly luminous but whitish green, which, in tending towards the blue, becomes more and more ' saturated '; so that greenish-blue must be the type of these hues. The *blue* is a green of moderate luminosity, and strongly ' saturated '; and *violet* is green very feebly luminous, but also ' saturated ' in a much higher degree than the normal. A violet strongly luminous is sufficient to induce this green, but a feeble violet, although very sensible to the normal eye, is black to the colour-blind in question."[1]

Hering describes this defect as *blue-yellow* blindness—the absence or insensitiveness of the blue-yellow substance being cited as the pre-disposing condition. This leaves red and green as definite colour sensations. Von Kries, who terms the two forms of red and green blindness *protanopia* and *deuteranopia* respectively, employs a similar designation to blue-yellow blindness, namely, *tritanopia*.

König's[2] observations on this type of partial colour-blindness (a study of five cases) seems to indicate that, like red-green blindness, blue-yellow blindness is a reduction form of colour-vision, in that matches, valid for the normal eye, are also accepted as correct by the tritanope. He locates the neutral point of the spectrum in the yellow, somewhere between 566 $\mu\mu$. and 570 $\mu\mu$. Colour matches were made with yellow and its complementary blue, and confusions found to exist between orange and reddish purple, yellowish green and bluish violet.

Donders, who has also examined a case of tritanopia, finds a large neutral band in the yellow and the spectrum shortened not only at the violet end but at the red end also.[3]

Stilling[4] has studied nine cases of blue-yellow blindness and his finding is that whether colour-blindness is congenital or acquired—very similar phenomena and characteristics make their appearance.

Abney[5] has only met with one genuine case of violet blindness, as he terms it. The case is remarkable because of the curious nomenclature employed. The only two

[1] Translation by Holmgren, *The Smithsonian Report*, 1877.
[2] *Sitzungen der Akademie der Wissenschaft*, 1897.
[3] *Ann. d'ocul.*, 1880, 34, 212, 1880.
[4] " Ueber Entstehung und Wesen der Anomalien des Farbensinnes." *Zeitschrift für Sinnesphysiologie*, 1910.
[5] *Colour-Vision*, 1895.

colours seen are red and *black*. All greens and blues are called black, the former " bright black," the latter " dark black." Yellow is described as white, and it is in this region that the neutral point occurs. It is worth noting that Miss Richardson's case saw blue as a dazzling white.

For a fairly extensive bibliography on this form of dichromasy consult Parsons' *An Introduction to the Study of Colour-Vision ;* *Further Advances in Physiology*, edited by Leonard Hill, London, 1909, an article on " Theories of Colour-Vision," by Greenwood.

3. *Total Colour-Blindness*

Monochromatic vision, or total colour-blindness, is not frequently encountered, only about eighty cases having been described in all. Its existence, however, has been proved beyond all dispute.

The totally colour-blind sees the spectrum as a colourless band differing only in luminosity ; no colour sensation at all is experienced. Such monochromats are in general painfully dazzled by bright light ; in fact, ordinary illumination of any kind is sometimes unbearable for them, but in dim light they can see fairly accurately. Usually, subjects suffering from such a defect also show symptoms of photophobia, nystagmus (or irregular movements of the eyes to and fro) and, in some cases, poor central vision.

It is difficult to imagine the visual sensations of such a colour-blind, but if we regard his case in not too detailed a manner, it is possible to compare his visual field to an engraving in contradistinction to a corresponding coloured picture.

A summary of the results of Hering, giving black and white equations of a typical colour-blind is very illuminating. They are quoted from Greenwood.[1]

[1] *Physiology of the Special Senses*, p. 108.

Hering's Case of Total Colour-Blindness

Coloured circle			Equally bright circle for colour-blind	
			White degrees	Black degrees
Bluish-red			13·0	347·0
Yellowish-red			5·5	354·5
Orange			37·0	323·0
Yellow			136·5	223·5
Arsenic green			228·0	132·0
Green			152·0	208·0
Greenish-blue			109·5	250·5
Ultramarine-blue			88·3	271·7
Violet			47·5	312·5

These Tables clearly show the difference in brightness which each colour in the spectrum has for the totally colour-blind. It is interesting to note that these equations are valid for the normal eye under conditions of dark adaptation.

There seem to exist two distinct forms of *achromatopia*, as it is sometimes called. In the one form, the region of maximal brightness is in the yellow, as in the normal eye, while in the other, the region of maximal brightness lies in the green. It is this second condition which appears to be so similar to the condition of the scotopic eye. In many cases an absolute central scotoma has been found to accompany the defect. This means that the fovea is totally blind not only to colour but to light sensations of any kind. The presence of nystagmus which accompanies so many cases of total colour-blindness, renders this fact difficult to establish, and it cannot be said conclusively that foveal blindness is present in all such cases. The statement can only be made that it occurs in many of the cases which have been recorded ; and further, as Parsons points out " Whether all cases have an absolute central scotoma or not, it is certain that foveal vision is very defective even as compared with parafoveal, as is admitted by Hess."[1]

Wilson in his *Researches on Colour-Blindness* states that total colour-blindness is rare, but that several well-marked cases are on record. He writes, " The most severe sufferer from colour-blindness may be expected to see as large and as perfect a rainbow or spectrum as others do, although to him it is colourless. The different bands, such as the bright yellow, the dark blue, and the intermediate red, will affect his eye differently in virtue of their different luminosity."

One of the cases collected by Wartmann goes back as far as 1684, and is quoted by Wilson. " A young woman, thirty-two or thirty-three years of age, came to consult Dr Dawbeney about her sight, which, though excellent in other respects, incapacitated her from appreciating any other colour than white and black, although she could often read for nearly a quarter of an hour in the greatest darkness." A family is referred to by Spurzheim, " all the members of which could only distinguish black and white." Three persons of one family, named Harris, are also referred to, " who distinguished in colours only tints of luminous intensity, calling all bright tints white, and all dull ones black."[2]

The following case described by Donders is quoted by Joy Jeffries.[3]

" Professor Donders reported an interesting case of

---

[1] *An Introduction to the Study of Colour-Vision*, p. 189.

[2] The original authorities for these statements are given in Taylor's *Scientific Memoirs*, 1846.

[3] *Colour-Blindness : its Dangers and its Detection*, p. 35. Footnote.

congenital total colour-blindness at the Heidelberg Ophthalmological Society, 1871 : An educated young man of twenty-one years of age was totally colour-blind. Strong light blinded him ; in moderate light he saw very well. He was myopic one-eighth, and read for hours without glasses. Out of doors, all glasses which absorbed light, without difference—even the brightest coloured ones—were pleasant to him, because they reduced the light. In the dioptric spectrum of a gas-lamp his brightest part was between the spectral lines, D and E, close to E : hence in greenish yellow. From here outwards towards the red end the light faded rapidly ; towards the violet, at first, slowly, then rapidly. By moderate illumination he lost less of the brightest of the spectrum on this side than towards the red end. With the polariscope, the complementary colours through the quartz plate appeared to him of the same colour. In turning the double refractive prism he had a maximum of brightness at every ninety degrees, or equality of brightness, as if the quartz plate was not there. He had the greatest difference when Donders himself saw purple and green ; equality, when he saw yellow and blue. Trials were also made with Chevreul's chromatic Circle."

These cases which have been quoted give a fairly clear account of the nature of the defect. One other case, studied by Hess and Hering[1], yields interesting features, and has attracted considerable attention.

Those cases in which foveal blindness occurs—blindness to light as well as to colour—tell in favour of certain theories. In the fovea there are no rods, only cones ; therefore, if total blindness occurs at the fovea, it seems to indicate that colourless light sensations are connected with

[1] *Psychological Review*, Vol. V, 1898 ; or *Pflüger's Archiv*, 71, 105.

the rods, since an area devoid of rods produces no light sensation whatever.

This fact seems to support the theories of König, von Kries, and Ladd-Franklin.   But different cases have been reported (at least three) in which there is no blindness at the fovea, implying, therefore, that in the fovea there must exist some form of apparatus capable of arousing light sensations.   If such facts are correct—as they undoubtedly are—they are unfavourable to all theories which state that cones produce sensations of colour, whereas rods are only concerned with colourless sensations.   It is Hering and Hess who have reported such cases in which no blindness at the fovea occurs.   These investigators, therefore, conclude that : " The hypothesis of König and von Kries, in accordance with which the totally colour-blind differ from those who have normal vision either by the absence or by the functionlessness of the cones, finds no support in our observations."[1]   Dr Ladd-Franklin, however, points out in the same article, that, although these cases do not support such theories, they do not, on the other hand, withdraw support from them.   In fact, Dr Ladd-Franklin states that three hypotheses suggest themselves, (a) that the foveæ of these three subjects contain not cones but rods : but that the rods are lacking in visual purple, a condition which has been established by Kühne as characterizing the rods in the immediate vicinity of the fovea.   (b) That the foveæ may contain undeveloped cones which are incapable of arousing any colour sensation, but which contain the same photochemical substance as the rods.   (c) That there must be no visual elements in the foveæ capable of performing any unction.

Dr Ladd-Franklin concludes that, " The result of this work of Hess and Hering, therefore, need not be anything

[1] *Psychological Review*, 1898, p. 503.

more than to force an upholder of this hypothesis[1] to
the assumption that there are two forms of total colour-
blindness, one (with nystagmus, foveal blindness, and
avoidance of high lights) due to a defective condition of
the cones, and the other (without those attendant
symptoms) due to some difficulty in the nerves of con-
duction in their receiving stations. And this latter form
is much the least frequent. It is certain that the totally
colour-blind boy whom Professor König had in his laboratory in the summer of 1894, had no vision in his fovea.
Of a group of small bright objects, he constantly lost
one out of sight ; and it was only necessary to stand in
front of him, and ask him to look at you, to see plainly
that in his effort to look you straight in the eye he was
obliged to turn his eyeball markedly to one side."[2]

4. *Acquired Colour-Blindness*

The study of acquired colour-blindness is a most interesting one. The individual has had normal colour vision,
but because of certain disease in the eye or brain his
colour-vision is impaired and he becomes to all intents
and purposes colour-blind. One feature which is common
to most cases of acquired colour-blindness is the presence
of some disease of the optic nerve. Acquired colour-
blindness, although apparently independent of defective
vision, invariably accompanies some other serious loss of
vision, either of form or of light. Sometimes the blindness
to colour only affects the fovea, and consequently only
central colour-vision is involved, just as frequently an
absolute central scotoma occurs in monochromatic
cases. The rest of the retina may have colour vision
unimpaired. A very common predisposing cause is over-

---

[1] Namely, that cones condition colour sensations, rods, colourless
sensations (Author's footnote).
[2] *Loc. cit.*

indulgence in tobacco. Red and green are the usual colours which are affected.[1] "Some will distinguish yellow, and very nearly all will distinguish blue with the centre of the eye. If a bright spectrum be thrown on the screen and a tobacco-blind person be requested to name the colours of the different parts pointed out to him, it is often the case that as his eyes follow the pointer he will tell you that in the extreme red he sees no light, but in the bright red he sees dull white. The bright yellow he will tell you is a pale yellow or white, according as his case is a moderate or a bad one ; the green he calls white, and the blue and violet he will designate correctly. At the same time that his eye is turned away to another colour, he will see the true colours of the part of the spectrum which he has just incorrectly named, but it will disappear again as he turns his eyes back again. This tells us that his sense of colour is apparently unaffected outside the diseased area." When testing such colour-blinds it is important that the colours shown be not too large, otherwise they will stimulate not only the diseased area, but the area outside it, and in consequence the colours will be accurately described or matched as the case may be.

Colour-blindness may be caused by an accident. Wilson[2] records the case of a physician who was thrown from his horse and who suffered concussion of the brain. "On recovering sufficiently to notice distinctly objects around him, he found that his perception of colours, which was formerly normal and acute, had become both weakened and perverted : and it has since continued so. . . . All coloured objects . . . now seem strange to him. The rainbow is quite destitute of hue,

---

[1] Abney, *Colour-Vision*, London, 1895, p. 142.
[2] *Researches on Colour-Blindness*, 1855, p. 39.

appearing as a white semicircle against the sky, or as a
lunar rainbow does to most normal eyes. This absence
of colour in the solar spectrum, however, is largely due
to the weakening of Mr B.'s colour-vision : for certain
of the tints of coloured objects held near to the eye are
well enough distinguished, especially yellow and blue.
Red and green are indistinguishable from each other. . . .
Whilst formerly a student in Edinburgh he was known as
an excellent anatomist ; now he cannot distinguish an
artery from a vein by its tint. He was previously fond
of sketching in colours ; but since his accident he has laid
it aside as a hopeless and unpleasant task. Flowers have
lost more than half their beauty for him, and he recalls
the shock which he received on first entering his garden
after his recovery, at finding that a favourite damask
rose had become in all its parts, petals, leaves, and stem,
of one uniform dull colour ; and that variegated flowers
had lost their characteristic tints."

Tyndall reports a case of Mr White Cooper.[1] It is
a most interesting case and, as Jeffries points out, contains
a word of warning.

" The sufferer was a sea captain, and, ten or twelve
years ago, was accustomed, when time lay heavy on his
hands, to occupy it by working at embroidery. Being
engaged one afternoon upon a piece of work of this description, and anxious to finish a flower (a red one, he believes)
he prolonged his labours until twilight fell, and he found
it difficult to select the suitable colours. To obtain more
light, he went into the companion, or entrance to the
cabin, and there continued his needlework. While thus
taxing his eyes, his power of distinguishing the colours
suddenly vanished. He went upon deck, hoping an

[1] Quoted in Jeffries, *Colour-Blindness : its Dangers and its Detection* ;
and in Edridge-Green, *Colour-Blindness and Colour-Perception.*

increase of light would restore his vision. In vain. From that time to the present he has remained colour-blind. Berlin worsted, with which he had been accustomed to work, he at once and correctly pronounced to be blue. He had a keen appreciation for this colour, and never made a mistake regarding it. Two bundles of worsted —one a light green, and the other a vivid scarlet—were next placed before him. He pronounced them to be both of the same colour. A difference in shade was perceptible ; but both to him were drab. A green glass and a red glass were placed side by side between him and the window ; he could discern no difference between the colours. A very dark green he pronounced to be black ; fruits, partly of a bright red and partly of a deep green, were pronounced to be of the same uniform colour. A cedar pencil and a stick of sealing-wax, placed side by side, were nearly alike. The former was rather brown ; the latter a drab. Electric light through a green glass, allowed to fall on a screen, gave him no colour, but only that portion of the screen was a little less intensely illuminated.

" Captain C. was assured that, previous to the circumstances related, he was a good judge of colours ; so that, pronouncing on any colour, he had an aid from memory not usually possessed by the colour-blind. Indeed, he had an opportunity of reviving his impression of red. A glass of this colour was placed before his eyes while he stood before the electric lamp. On establishing the light, he at once exclaimed, ' That is red ! ' He appeared delighted to renew his acquaintance with this colour, and he declared that he had not seen it for several years. The glass was then held near the light, while he went to a distance ; but in this case no colour was manifest ; neither was any colour seen when a gas-lamp was regarded through the same glass. The intense action due to proximity to the electric light appeared to produce the effect. Captain C.'s interest in this experiment was increased by the fact that the Portland light, which he had occasion to observe, has been recently changed from green to red ; but he has not been able to recognize this change. The fare in the fore-cabin of a vessel of his own, which he now commands, happens to be sixpence ; and he is often reminded by the passengers that he has not returned their change. The reason is, that he confounds a sixpence with a half-sovereign, both being to him the same colour. A short time age he gave a sovereign to a waterman, believing it to be a shilling."

An instructive instance of acquired colour-blindness is recorded by Köllner.[1] He watched the progress of the disorder from normal colour-vision to complete colour defect. He found that two stages can be distinguished. First in the early stage, the defect somewhat resembles the conditions of anomalous trichromatism. But to begin with, yellow and red are distinguished, although yellow and green are confused.

In the second stage,[2] " and final stage all the colours from red to the neutral band in the blue-green are confused, and distinguished only by differences in brightness."

Where the defect is caused by tobacco or by a drug such as santonin, it is progressive in character, and at first may be indicated only by a failing of the visual faculties. No loss of colour perception may be noticed, and usually the disease is far advanced before a defect in colour becomes evident. Such defect, however, unlike the other forms of colour-blindness, is curable, and absence of the cause restores colour-vision to normal. It will be evident that tests for colour-blinds, when for practical purposes, should

[1] " Zur Entstehung der erworbenen Rotgrünblindheit," *Zeitschrift für Sinnesphysiologie*, 1910.
[2] *Psychological Bulletin*, 1911, Article by Hayes.

be instituted at regular intervals in order to detect any progressive cases of colour anomaly.

Artificial colour-blindness may be produced by fatiguing the eye for certain colours ; for example, if red-blindness is induced, then scarlet flowers will appear black, and pink flowers sky-blue, as in the experiments carried out by G. J. Burch.[1]

[1] See Greenwood's *Physiology of the Special Senses*.

CHAPTER II

COLOUR THEORIES WITH SPECIAL REFERENCE TO COLOUR-BLINDNESS

In all theories it seems more or less agreed that colour-blindness is a reduction system of normal colour vision. Again and again it has been found that equations valid for the normal eye are equally valid for the colour-blind eye. This points to the conclusion that the dichromate lacks something which the normal eye has—but has nothing which the normal eye does not possess.

1. *Young-Helmholtz Theory*

(The Three Components Theory)

This theory first propounded in 1801 by Thos. Young and resuscitated in 1860 by Helmholtz is one of the most important.

The colour sensations are reduced to three fundamental colours, red, green, and violet, corresponding to which there are three nerve fibres in the retina—now replaced by three photochemical substances.

Stimulation of the first fibre produces red, of the second, green, and of the third, violet. But homogeneous light excites all three in different proportions according to the wave lengths.

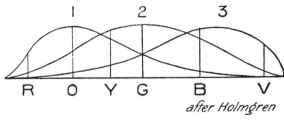

FIG. I

The three curves represent the proportional stimulation of each set of nerve fibres with pure light. (1) is red nerve fibre, (2) green, (3) violet.

Red.   Stimulates strongly the red, less the other two.   *Sensation is Red.*

Yellow. Stimulates moderately the red and green, feebly the violet.   *Sensation is Yellow.*

Green. Stimulates strongly the green, much less the other two.   *Sensation is Green.*

Blue.   Stimulates moderately the green and violet, feebly the red.   *Sensation is Blue.*

Violet. Stimulates strongly the violet, feebly the other two.   *Sensation is Violet.*

Equally strong stimulation of all the fibres gives the sensation of white. Absence of stimulation gives the sensation of black.

The red now adopted as primitive is a carmine red (a red bluer than the extreme red of the spectrum), the green, a yellowish green, and the third element an ultramarine blue.

Colour-Blindness

According to this theory the partial colour-blinds may
be divided into the following classes :

1. Partial colour-blindness, in which one of the three
   fundamental sensations is completely absent.
   A. Red-blindness.
   B. Green-blindness.
   C. Violet-blindness.

2. Incomplete colour-blindness, where one or all of the
   three fundamental elements are inferior in
   excitability.

Red-Blindness

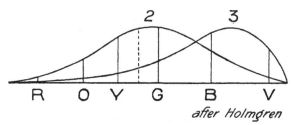

after Holmgren

Fig. II

In red-blindness, the colour sensations of the individual
are reduced to green and violet.

Red.   Appears as a saturated green of very feeble
            intensity.
Feeble Red. Does not sufficiently stimulate any of the
            fibres ; therefore it appears black.
Yellow.   Appears as a saturated green and intensely
            luminous, " and as it constitutes the precisely
            saturated and very intense shade of that colour,
            it can be understood how the red-blind select

E

the name of that colour, and call all those tints that are properly speaking green, yellow."[1]

Green. Appears as a more intense but whitish shade of the same colour as yellow and red.

White. Is composed of the two elementary colours and appears blue-grey to normal vision.

The colours between green and blue are seen, therefore, as grey. The rest of the spectrum appears blue or violet.

Green-Blindness

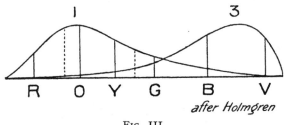

after Holmgren

Fig. III

In the case of the absence of the green element—the colour system is derived from the other two elements, red and violet.

Red. Stimulates strongly the red fibre and faintly the violet one. It appears to the green-blind as a strongly saturated red.

Orange. Also a saturated red.

Yellow. A more intensely luminous red than spectral red.

Green. Is the grey of the colour-blind because it is composed of equal parts of red and violet.

Blue. Is an intense violet.

---

[1] Quoted by Holmgren. See *Smithsonian Report*, 1877.

This explanation of the two common types of red- and green-blindness was accepted for some time, and experiments which were carried out seemed to fit in with the theoretical hypotheses. The first objection to the theory as an explanation of colour-blindness was raised by Edmund Rose, who, from his own personal experience, based on observation of colour-blinds, found the theory to be incompatible with fact. He found that both types of colour-blinds declared their fundamental sensations to be yellow and blue. Helmholtz noted Rose's results, but thought they were insufficient to alter his theory, although he admitted that, " in the case of congenital colour-blindness, it might well be imagined that the activity of the nerve fibres might not be removed, but that the intensity curves of the three kinds of light-sensitive elements might change, whereby a much greater variability in the effect of objective colours on the eye might arise."[1]

John Aitken, F.R.S., of Falkirk, in a paper on " Colour Sensation "[2] suggested that " the nerves might be so constructed that the red nerves might be sensitive to all the rays to which the green nerves are sensitive," so that, both nerves being excited by either red or green rays, " the sensation produced would be what we call yellow."

Leber,[3] in 1873, published results which seemed to confirm the view that yellow was the sensation of the dichromic, because the red and green fibres were equally stimulated. This explanation was later adopted by Fick,[4] and König, in 1886, expounded the same view at a meeting of the British Association in Birmingham.

[1] *Handbuch der Physiologischen Optik*, 2nd Edition.
[2] *Scottish Society of Arts*, 1872. Quoted from Pole's Article in *Transactions of the Royal Society of Edinburgh*, 1893.
[3] Zehender's *Klinische Monatsblätter für Augenheilkunde*, Vol. XI, 1873.
[4] Hermann's *Handbuch der Physiologie*, Vol, III, Part 1. 1879.

Helmholtz, in 1892, in the second edition of his *Physiological Optics*, confirms this new modification of the theory, and further points out that the former division into red and green-blinds is no longer advisable. " One of the greatest stones of stumbling for years past has been the division, consequent on the ' old ' explanation, of dichromic patients into the two theoretically distinct classes of ' red-blind ' and ' green-blind.' It is obvious that this division naturally disappears when the old explanation is abandoned; but Helmholtz takes pains to show geometrically that his new theory gives no place for such a division. And he, moreover, expresses the opinion that such a division does not seem to have been fully justified by observation."[1]

According to this new explanation red-blindness would be explained thus :

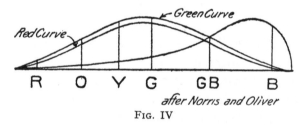

FIG. IV

The red element has become similar in sensitivity to the green element.

The spectrum consists of yellow and blue, but the yellow begins not in the red but in the orange. Blue-green excites all three elements and therefore is seen as grey ; the neutral band therefore lies towards the violet end of the spectrum. The red and green curves, equally excited, give sensations of yellow.

[1] *Philosophical Magazine*, Article by W. Pole, " Helmholtz Theories," 35, 1893.

Green-Blind

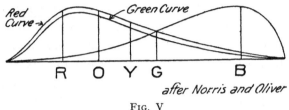

FIG. V

The green element has become similar in sensitivity to the red element.

The spectrum is seen as shades of yellow and blue.

The green excites all three elements and therefore will be seen as grey. (Note the difference from the case above, where the neutral band lay in the blue-green.)

Again, red and blue are stimulated equally at this point, giving the purple of the normal eye ; therefore, purple is equal to grey, which in turn is seen as green.

2. *McDougall's Theory*

McDougall has modified the Young-Helmholtz theory.[1] He accepts the three fundamental colours, red, green and blue, but adds an independent mechanism for white having its retinal seat in the rods. In the first place, he bases his theories on a large number of observations carried out on the fading and " mutual inhibitions " of visual images. Secondly, he argues that the hypothesis of a special black-exciting process, such as is postulated with Hering's theory, is unnecessary. McDougall, therefore, adopts the duplicity theory of von Kries. He writes, " von Kries has brought together evidence that makes it appear in the highest degree probable that the

[1] See *Mind*, N.S., Vol. X, 1901.

rods are the retinal elements of an independent white apparatus, which functions alone in the normal eye when affected by light of low intensity only, and in the monochromatic eye. This view of the functions of the rods had been suggested thirty years before to Max Schultze by his studies in comparative histology. This hypothesis of an independent white-exciting function of the rods must then be taken up into and incorporated with Young's theory, and then, when this is done, the difficulty in representing the development of the visual processes in terms of this theory at once fades away."[1]

McDougall thus assumes a separate retino-cerebral apparatus for each of the three photopic colours of red, green and blue, and for the scotopic white element. He further assumes that each eye has its own set of four such systems quite independent of the other. The sensation of black is experienced when " complete fading " occurs and the visual cortex is at rest.

Colour-Blindness

His explanation of colour-blindness follows from his theory of the evolution of the colour sense. Vision begins first, and exists in the lower animals, as monochromatic, varying only in brightness, and similar to our white or grey sensation. The first stage is the differentiation of the rays of light of the warm and cold ends of the spectrum. The cold rays, in addition to setting free a white-exciting substance, would begin to set free " a substance that by the excitement of a concurrently differentiated retino-cerebral apparatus would add the sensation of blue to that of white."[2] Similarly, the warm rays would produce a sensation of yellow. If mixed light stimulates the retina at this stage of development, all three systems will

[1] *Ibid.*, p. 211–2.   [2] *Ibid.*

be excited. McDougall points out that it would be advantageous for the yellow and blue to fuse and form white and thereby reinforce the sensation of white caused by the excitation of the older apparatus. If yellow and blue fused to give a new sensation—the result of stimulation by mixed light would be a sensation composed of this new colour added to white—the pure sensation of white would then be lost for ever. All that would be possible would be yellow and blue and a yellowish blue probably.

The peripheral zone of the retina is still a relic of this primitive stage of monochromatic vision, while the totally colour-blind are cases of a total reversion to " this remote ancestral condition."

The middle zone of the retina shows the second stage of differentiation in which yellow, blue, and white are all that are experienced, and the " frequent cases of bichromatic vision, in which yellow and blue and white seem to be the only sensations that can be aroused by stimulation of the retina, are cases of reversion to or arrested development in this more recent ancestral condition."

McDougall, tracing the stage of evolution further, shows how, for advantageous reasons, the differentiation would next proceed in the region of the yellow, giving rise to the sensations of red and green. These, when stimulated simultaneously, fuse in a yellow sensation ; otherwise the primitive white and the original yellow will be lost. As the red and green developed (and the development takes place from the *fovea centralis* outwards), yellow would disappear from the central region, just as white itself no longer is found in the fovea. The white, however, remains in the other parts of the retina, probably because it assists vision in dim illumination.

This view, McDougall claims, especially when it is remembered that the rods are the end organs for the white apparatus, brings the Young theory, as he prefers to call it, into harmony with all the known facts, especially with regard to those of colour-blindness.

3. Hering's Theory

(The Opponent Colours Theory)

The Hering[1] theory rivals the Young-Helmholtz in importance. Hering bases his theory on six elementary colours, elementary so far as introspection can discover. These are red, green, yellow, blue, white, black. Red, green, yellow, and blue are the toned or bright (*bunte*) colours ; white and black are the toneless colours. The toneless colours can be arranged in a graded series from the most intense white to the deepest black, forming, when combined in different proportions, various shades of grey ; the toned colours can be arranged in a circular series with the four elementary colours forming four divisions. The colours, therefore, can be arranged in two pairs, yellow and blue forming one pair ; red and green the other. We cannot pass directly from yellow to blue, we have to pass through green, a member of the other pair. In other words, we cannot have a reddish green nor a yellowish blue. The yellow may combine with the red and form a new compound colour in which both elements are recognizable, or with green and form a yellow-green, but it cannot combine with the other member of the same pair, blue, and form a compound colour. For, no matter what proportions of yellow and blue are combined, no new hue will appear ; the mixture will appear either yellow or blue, except where the two

[1] *Zur Lehre vom Lichtsinne*, 1878 : *Zur Erklärung der Farbenblindheit, aus der Theorie der Gegenfarben*, 1880.

colours are neutralized, and then neither colour will be recognizable. These complementary colours forming a pair are, therefore, opposed or antagonistic colours.

Corresponding to these two pairs of antagonistic colours, there exist two elementary systems somewhere in the retino-cerebral apparatus, one of which gives rise to red and green, the other to yellow and blue. A third system gives the colourless sensations of black and white. The physiological action of a colour and its complementary is antagonistic. Each of the substances can undergo a building up or an anabolic process, and a breaking down or a katabolic process.

Red	is caused by	katabolism	,,	red-green	apparatus
Orange	,,	{katabolism	,,	red-green	,,
		{katabolism	,,	yellow-blue	,,
Yellow	,,	katabolism	,,	yellow-blue	,,
Green	,,	anabolism	,,	red-green	,,
Blue	,,	anabolism	,,	yellow-blue	,,
Violet	,,	{katabolism	,,	red-green	,,
		{anabolism	,,	yellow-blue	,,
White	,,	katabolism	,,	white-black	,,
Black	,,	anabolism	,,	white-black	,,

In most kinds of stimulation all three systems are set in action and the resultant sensation depends upon the relative amount of excitation of each substance. Thus orange is composed of red and yellow, and in Hering's terminology we should say that orange has a red " value " (*Valenz*) and a yellow " value." Further, all spectral colours contain white, so that each colour has a white " value " in addition. This white is most distinct in the yellow and the yellow-green. All coloured lights, except the four primary colours, have therefore three values corresponding to their action on the three different substances. All rays from the extreme red end of the spectrum have in addition an effect on the yellow process as far as the pure or fundamental green. These rays are said to have a yellow value. All rays from the green to the violet end of the spectrum affect the blue process —they are said to have a blue value. The yellow is so weak at the beginning of the spectrum that the red overpowers it, and the ultimate sensation experienced is red—the yellow is invisible to the normal eye. The four divisions of the spectrum may thus be represented :

First division contains Red and Yellow and White.
Pure Yellow   ,,   Yellow and White.
Second division ,,   Yellow and Green and White.
Pure Green   ,,   Green and White.
Third division   ,,   Green and Blue and White.
Pure Blue   ,,   Blue and White.
Fourth division   ,,   Blue and Red and White.

The spectrum, therefore, can be divided according to the excitation of the yellow-blue substances, and we get yellow in the first half, blue in the second half ; these two divided by pure green with a white value.

Hering substituted for his former explanation of luminosity as wholly due to the black-white component, the theory of " the specific brightness of colours." Certain colours possess an inherent brightness or darkness of their own. The brightness of a colour sensation depends, therefore, on two causes : (1) on the inherent brightness (or darkness) of the colour itself; (2) on the amount of excitation of the white-black process. The warm colours, red and yellow, possess an inherent brightness (*Eigenhelligkeit*) ; the cold colours, green and blue, possess an inherent darkness (*Eigendunkelheit*). " A toned colour may generally be regarded as made up of four fundamental components, two toned and two tone-free (white and black). It is only in colours of the tone of a primary that a single-toned component is present. In any red-yellow colour, *e.g.*, orange, we have, therefore, to distinguish three fundamental components (red, yellow, white), and one dark (black) ; in any green-blue, on the other hand, three dark (green, blue, black), and one bright (white). The red-blue and the green-yellow colours would contain two bright and two dark fundamental components.

" From what has been said, the following rules can be deduced :

" If two colours of equal tone and equal purity differ in brightness, this is due to a difference in their black-white components.

" Two colours differing in tone may, notwithstanding equal degrees of purity and equality as regards their black-white components, differ in brightness.

" With equality of conditions as to the black-white components, a yellow, a red, or a yellow-red colour is so much the brighter, a blue, a green, or a blue-green so much the darker, the more distinct the colour tone in comparison with the black-white components."[1]

Colour-Blindness

Red-green blindness is due to the absence of the red-green substance. As we have already seen, if the red and green elements are removed, the sensations of yellow, blue, black and white still remain. The sensations of the red-green colour-blinds are accordingly yellow and blue. Red, orange, yellow and some of the green will

[1] Quoted from Greenwood, *Physiology of the Special Senses.*

appear as yellows of different degrees of saturation; part of the green and blue and violet will appear as blues of different degrees of saturation. The pure green will be colourless.

The peripheral zone of the retina, according to Hering, shows the same conditions as in colour-blindness. In the outermost zone of the retina, as in total colour-blindness, only the white-black substance is present. Red-green blindness corresponds to the middle zone of the retina, where yellow and blue are the only colours experienced. The investigations which Hess[1] has carried out along these lines have given strong confirmation of Hering's views.

Hering's greatest difficulty has been to account for the two varieties of red-green colour-blindness. Undoubtedly both types see yellow and blue in the spectrum. But they vary in regard to the region of the yellow in which the point of maximal brightness occurs. Hering explained this difference as due to differences of pigmentation of the *macula* and lens, and offered the same explanation to account for the differences in normal vision of anomalous trichromates. The yellow pigment in the *macula* absorbs the warm end of the spectrum very little, is at its maximum in the yellow-green region, and diminishes in action towards the cold end of the spectrum.

Hering, in 1885,[2] examined a number of cases and found he could divide them into two groups. One group matched spectral red with spectral blue in the ratio of 1·15 : 1, the other group in the ratio of 7 to 1. He found the position of pure green to differ in the two groups—the green requiring to be of greater wave-length in the case of the first group. In colourless mixtures of

[1] *Pflüger's Archiv*, Vol, LXXI, p. 105, sqq.
[2] *Lotos*, 6 N.F.

red and bluish-green, greenish-yellow and violet, and yellow and blue, the first group required larger quantities of the shorter wave-length component. The first group was said to be relatively yellow-sighted, the second group relatively blue-sighted, the distinction being based on their responsiveness to these colours. Hering examined two marked cases of individual variation in pigmentation —Professor Biedermann and Dr Singer. Professor Biedermann, with little macular pigmentation, he termed relatively yellow-sighted ; Dr Singer, with greater pigmentation, he termed relatively blue-sighted. Hering therefore suggested that the two classes of red-green colour-blindness were extreme cases of yellow- and blue-sightedness, combined with greater or lesser pigmentation of the *macula*. The protanopes or scoterythrous group would be regarded as relatively blue-sighted (or blue anomalous) ; the deuteranopes or photerythrous would be regarded as relatively yellow-sighted.

If the explanation is correct, one would expect to find gradation cases—passing gradually from protanopia to deuteranopia—but such does not seem to be the case. Von Kries and Abney, by experimentation, have shown that the basis of differentiation between scoterythrous and photerythrous cannot be a physical one. Tschermak, a staunch adherent of Hering's theory, is also inclined to give up this explanation.[1]

Dr Rivers, however, states that "the variations of pigmentation may be discontinuous ; and in the absence of direct investigation of the question the existence of two distinct groups by no means destroys the validity of the proposed explanation. It seems probable to Hering that there is a relation between macular (and lens) pigmentation and development of the colour sense.

[1] Tschermak, *Ergebnisse der Physiologie*, 1902.

In cases of red-green blindness, it seemed as if the group with more pigmentation (yellow-sighted or photerythrous) had a more highly developed blue-yellow sense, and Hering supposes that the shortening of the spectrum in the scoterythrous group may be due to weakness of the yellow sensation."[1]

4. Müller's Theory

Müller is an exponent of the Hering theory, and has suggested some modifications.[2] He accepts as fundamental the colours red, yellow, green and blue of Hering and the white-black apparatus. These four chromatic processes and the two achromatic processes are at the periphery ; but in addition to these there are six central values. The red process excites the red, yellow and white values ; the yellow process excites the yellow, green and white ; the green process excites the green, blue, and black ; the blue process excites the blue, red and black. The yellow process excites the red and the yellow processes, thereby exciting the red, green, yellow and white values. The red and green neutralize one another, leaving the sensation of yellow.

Müller substituted a reversible chemical process for Hering's antagonistic processes of anabolism and katabolism.

Müller was dissatisfied with Hering's explanation of the two types of red-green colour-blindness and gives the following explanation. "The red light of the spectrum, he assumes, besides its effect on the red-green substance, may have also an effect on the yellow-blue substance, and it may even have two such effects—it may act upon it, in

[1] Article in Schäfer's *Text-book of Physiology*, p. 1118-9.
[2] *Zeitschrift für Psychologie und Physiologie der Sinnesorgane*, 10, 1896 ; 14, 1897.

the first place, directly, by producing out of the decomposition of the red-green substance some one or more of the constituents of the yellow material (with which, in the original form of the hypothesis, red light had nothing to do). The first type of the red-green blind—those formerly called red-blind—are totally lacking in the red-green substance ; these are the typical yellow-blue visioned. But the second type—those formerly called green-blind—see yellow in the place of both red and green for some totally different reason—either because the nerve fibres which conduct the retinal excitation are not of the normal constitution, or because some still other constituent which is usually found already prepared in the retina is now absent. In this fashion it will be seen that the so-called red-blind lack all the *indirect* effect of the light of the spectrum upon the yellow-blue substance, while that indirect effect still persists for the green-blind."[1] Ladd-Franklin regards this explanation as complicated and far-fetched.

5. *Ladd-Franklin's Theory*

(The Molecular Dissociation Theory)

This theory assumes that the colour sense in the earliest stage of its existence was restricted to grey only, which includes the whole range of colourless sensations. The sensation of grey is produced by the decomposition of a grey molecule. The decomposition of the molecule sets free a chemical substance which acts upon the retinal nerve endings and so a sensation is experienced. The molecule consists of a firm inner core to which is loosely attached an outer range of atoms. These atoms are

---

[1] *Psychological Review*, Vol. VI, Article by C. Ladd-Franklin.

" torn off " in decomposition and the sensation ensues. The cause of the " tearing off " of the atoms is the ether vibrations which are in the visible spectrum. The middle part of the spectrum has a more powerful effect on the atoms, as is shown by the sensations of the totally colour-blind.

This grey substance exists both in the rods and in the cones. In the rods it still exists in an undifferentiated condition, so that " it goes to pieces all at once under the influence of light of any kind."[1] In the cones a differentiation has taken place and decomposition takes place in different stages. But the complete decomposition of the molecules in both rods and cones excites sensations of white or grey. " For black, the theory supposes that, in the interest of a continuous field of view, objects which reflect no light at all upon the retina have correlated with them a definite non-light sensation—that of black."[2]

The colour molecule appears at the second stage of development. The outer range of atoms in the cones segregate into two groups, having different vibration rates ; " one fitted to be shaken to pieces by light from the warm end of the spectrum, and the other by light from the cold end of the spectrum,"[3] and the two sensations of yellow and blue are experienced : " in a third stage of development, the yellow-producing constituent is in its turn broken up into two parts of such different internal vibrative periods that they respond respectively to the red light and green light of the spectrum."[4] The red and green colours are not complementary. If the red and green atoms are decomposed

[1] *Psychological Review*, Vol. III.
[2] Quoted from Woodworth, *Psychology : a Study of Mental Life*, p. 223.
[3] *Psychological Review*, Vol. VI.
[4] *Ibid.*, Vol. VI.

together, they revert to the more primitive yellow response. Similarly, when the yellow and blue atoms are decomposed together, they revert to the more primitive white or grey sensation. When all three, yellow, red and green are stimulated, complete decomposition takes place, and the original grey sensation results. These reversions must take place below the level of consciousness, for yellow does not appear to be composed of red and green nor white of yellow and blue. The combination will take place probably within the retina and be of the nature of a chemical union of some kind.

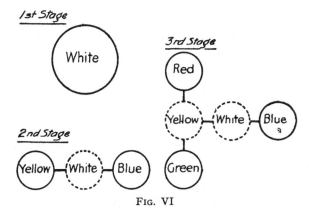

FIG. VI

This theory assumes three fundamental colours, red, green and blue, out of which all others arise by combination; it also recognizes the four primal colours, red, green, blue, yellow, each unlike the other three. A compound colour such as blue-green is formed in the following way. The blue rays " tear off " from the molecules the atoms corresponding to the vibrations of the blue rays, and the green rays " tear " from the molecules the atoms whose vibration rates are coincident with the green rays, and the resultant sensation is blue-green.

F

The first stage corresponds to the sensation experienced in the peripheral zone of the normal eye ; the second stage corresponds to the middle yellow-blue zone; the third stage to complete vision such as in the fovea.

The grey substance in the rods can be decomposed by a single-colour stimulus—but the grey substance in the cones requires a compound-colour stimulus before the sensation of grey can be experienced. As we have already seen, stimulation of the cones by a single colour only causes partial decomposition and a colour sensation is produced.

The rod-pigment or visual purple which is " not the substance whose chemical decomposition affects the optical nerve-ends "[1] is a secondary means for securing adaptation to a faint light, and not directly a vision-producing substance at all. It acts by absorbing (for the purpose of reinforcing faint light vision) a large amount of the light which usually passes entirely through the transparent rods and cones to be lost in the choroid coat . . . it is adapted to aiding vision in the gloomy depths of forests because green light is the light which it absorbs, and fishes, which alone, of all vertebrates, have a rod pigment of a distinctly different colour, are exactly fitted for utilizing the last rays of the light which penetrate deep into the waters of the sea."[2]

Colour-Blindness

Dr Ladd-Franklin regards colour-blindness as an atavistic condition. In total colour-blindness the grey molecule has remained undifferentiated and grey is the sole sensation of which the retina is capable. In red-green blindness the second stage of development is permanent. The grey molecule has become differentiated into yellow

[1] *Ibid.*, Vol. V. [2] *Ibid.*, Vol. VI.

and blue, but no further differentiation has taken place. Yellow and blue, therefore, are the only two colours which are visible to the red-green colour-blind. "It is as if red-vision had fallen out and green-vision had been turned into yellow-vision for the one sort ; and for the other sort it is as if green-vision had fallen out and yellow-vision had taken the place of red-vision."[1]

6. *Schenck's Theory*

Schenck's theory[2] seems to be along somewhat similar lines. He is, however, an advocate of the Young-Helmholtz theory which Ladd-Franklin does not claim to be. He recognizes five simple sensations, red, green, yellow, blue and white, but only three of these are fundamental, red, green and blue, which correspond physiologically to three " visual substances." He explains the development of the colour sense as starting from a sensation of white, which is conditioned by a visual substance which belongs to the cones only and which corresponds very closely to a similar substance in the scotopic visual substance of the rods. The white substance becomes differentiated into two substances, giving sensations of yellow and blue respectively which, when simultaneously excited, determine a reversion to the primitive sensation of white. Ultimately the yellow substance becomes differentiated into red and green which, when equally and simultaneously stimulated, arouse the sensation of yellow. White and yellow accordingly have no simple physiological counterparts.

Schenck assumes that each of the three visual sub-

[1] *Ibid.*, Vol. VI.
[2] *Arch. f. d. ges. Physiol.*, cxviii, 129, 1907.

stances has two parts.[1]   One part acts as a receiver for the stimulus [a stimulus-receptor (*Reizempfänger*) or, as has been suggested by Richarz, a kind of optical resonator] and this determines the luminosity of the sensation ; a second part, which determines the nature and intensity of the sensation, is set into activity by the receptor.   This is called the sensation-stimulator (*Empfindungserreger*), and according to its excitation, which is dependent on the amount of energy set free by the stimulus-receptor, the luminosity of the resultant sensation is determined.

Colour-Blindness

The red substance has a special stimulus-receptor and sensation-stimulator, and so have the green and blue ; the red for long waves, the green for medium waves and the blue for short waves.   The amount of energy set free by the green receptor, for example, goes directly to the green stimulator, with which it is associated physiologically, and no energy is diverted along any other channels.

In red-green colour-blindness, however, a difference occurs.   The blue receptor acts as before for the short-waved stimulus; the red and green are not differentiated, and objective light acts on the red or green receptor or on both, but they in turn are connected indiscriminately with the two corresponding receptors; the resultant sensation therefore is always that of yellow.   Schenck regards red-green colour-blindness as a case of arrested development, in which the final differentiation of yellow into red and green has not taken place.   In deuteranopia the three receptors and stimulators seem to be present, but the association between them has not become established in the case of the red and green visual

[1] See Parsons, *An Introduction to the Study of Colour-Vision*, p. 286.

substance. In protanopia, on the other hand, the receptor of the red visual substance is absent—although the stimulator is present. This means that long-waved light would cause no sensation at all in the case of red blindness, but medium-waved light would stimulate the receptor of the green visual substance, which would distribute its energy indiscriminately between the red and the green stimulators causing a sensation of yellow.

7. Edridge-Green's Theory

Professor Edridge-Green's theory assumes that visual purple is the sole visual substance. Visual purple is to be found in the rods only, and the rods are concerned merely with the formation of visual purple and take no part in visual sensations. (This is contrary to the strong evidence adduced in favour of his duplicity theory by von Kries and also by others who hold that the rods are the visual organs for scotopic vision.)[1]

Light rays impinge on the retina, setting free the visual purple from the rods, and a photograph or optogram is formed on the retina. The decomposition of the visual purple or rhodopsin stimulates the ends of the cones, setting up a visual impulse which is transmitted to the brain via the optic nerve. " In the impulse itself we have the physiological basis of the sensation of light, and in the quality of the impulse the physiological basis of the sensation of colour. The impulse being conveyed along the optic nerve to the brain, stimulates the visual centre, causing a sensation of light, then passing on to the colour-perceiving centre, causes a sensation of colour.

[1] The experiment, carried out by Ladd-Franklin and Ebbinghaus, reported in *Nature*, Vol. XLVIII, p. 517, seems further conclusive evidence against this view.

But though the impulses vary in character according to the wave-length of the light causing them, the retino-cerebral apparatus is not able to discriminate between the character of adjacent stimuli, not being sufficiently developed for the purpose. At most, seven distinct colours are seen, whilst others see, in proportion to the development of their colour-perceiving centre, only 6, 5, 4, 3 or 2. In the degrees of colour-blindness just preceding total, only the colours at the extremes of the spectrum are recognized as different, the remainder of the spectrum appearing grey."[1]

In the fovea there are cones only and no rods, therefore there is an absence of visual purple in the fovea. Edridge-Green claims, however, from direct observation and on entoptic grounds, that there are four canals or depressions leading into the fovea which conduct the visual purple from the rods into the centre of acutest vision. He and Devereux Marshall examined the retinas of two monkeys which had been kept in a dark room for forty-eight hours beforehand, and they claimed that the visual purple could be seen between the cones in the fovea.[2] Their observations, however, have not been confirmed—in fact, have been contradicted by Kühne and Nettleship. Entoptically the visual purple in the canals can be seen, on waking in the morning, as a rose-red star projected against a dull white surface, such as the ceiling. This observation of Edridge-Green confirms that previously made by Tait[3] and Boll.

" It is difficult to say at present exactly how the visual purple acts as a stimulus transformer, but this is because so many plausible hypotheses immediately occur to us. It is very probable that light acting upon the visual

[1] *Hunterian Lectures on Colour-Vision and Colour-Blindness*, p. 10, *sqq.*
[2] *Transactions of the Ophthalmological Society*, 1902, p. 300.
[3] *Proceedings of the Royal Society of Edinburgh*, 7, 605, 1869.

purple is, according to its wave-length, absorbed by particular atoms or molecules, the amplitude of their vibrations being increased. These vibrations may cause corresponding vibrations in certain discs of the outer segments of the cones, which seem especially constructed to take up vibrations. We know that when light falls on the retina it causes an electric current. We know how the telephone is able, through electricity, to convey waves of sound, and something similar may be present in the eye, the apparatus being especially constructed for vibrations of small wave-length. The current of electricity set up by light may cause the sensation of light, and the vibrations of the atoms or molecules the sensations of colour."[1]

He further points out that two processes are continually going on in the visual purple, as in all vital processes ; a katabolic or breaking-down process of the visual purple by light and an anabolic or building-up process by the pigment cells and rods.

" The retina, therefore, corresponds to a layer of photochemical liquid in which there are innumerable wires, each connected with a galvanometer. When light falls upon a portion of this fluid, the needle of the galvanometer corresponding to the nearest wire is deflected. The wires correspond to the separate fibres of the optic nerve, and the galvanometers to the visual centres of the brain."[2]

Colour-Blindness

Edridge-Green bases his theory of the evolution of the colour sense on his theory of psycho-physical units. A psycho-physical series is a physical series as it appears

[1] *Hunterian Lectures on Colour-Vision and Colour-Blindness*, p. 21, *sqq.*
[2] *Ibid.*, p. 23.

to the mind.   In colour the physical series is represented
by the solar spectrum, but the psycho-physical series
differs greatly with individuals.   The majority of
individuals are able to distinguish six different colours
in the spectrum, red, orange, yellow, green, blue and
violet, and they are said to have six psycho-physical
units.   The colour sense has gradually evolved by the
increase of the number of psycho-physical units.

At first no colour is seen—the spectrum appears as
different shades of grey.   The first differentiation of
colour will be that of the two physical stimuli which
are most unlike.   The spectrum then will appear all grey
but with a tinge of red at one end and a tinge of violet
at the other end.   As the colour sense improves, the
red and violet will gradually invade the grey band of
the spectrum, until they may meet in the centre.   " It is
obvious that all the colours of the normal-sighted which
are included in the coloured portion of the spectrum will
be seen alike and may be represented by that colour of
the normal-sighted which corresponds to the centre of
this coloured portion.   What are the two colours seen
when the whole of the grey has disappeared ?   The
colour will be represented by that colour which in the
normal-sighted corresponds to the centre of each of the
two colours.   According to the theory, these centre
points ought to correspond to the centres of the two
halves of the physical series.   The two colours should be
complementary to each other.   It is evident that
these complementaries must be those which are closest
to each other as far as the spectrum is concerned.
The   complementaries   which   are   adjacent   to   each
other are yellow and blue."[1]   Such cases are called
" dichromics."

[1] *Colour-Blindness and Colour-Perception*, pp. 34–5.

In the next stage of evolution, a third colour appears between the other two, namely, green. Such cases are " trichromics," and can see accordingly red, green and violet. They do not see yellow and blue and are continually in difficulty with them. Yellow is the next colour to appear between the red and the green and those who can see four colours in the spectrum (red, yellow, green, violet) are termed " tetrachromics." In the next stage of evolution the colours seen are red, yellow, green, blue, violet—these are the " pentachromics." Orange is the sixth colour to be recognized and thus we get the " hexachromics " or normal group to which the majority of individuals belong. The highest development yet reached is that of the " heptachromic " who can distinguish seven colours in the spectrum—the additional colour being indigo. " This order is not in agreement with careful observations on thresholds of colour-visibility by Abney and Festing and by Abney and Watson."[1]

Colour-blindness is atavistic and all stages are represented among colour-blinds. The " dichromics " correspond to the class usually termed " dichromates." The Anomalous Trichromates include the three, four and five unit class of Edridge-Green.

Colour-blindness can be divided into two classes. In the first class there is a defect of light perception as well as a colour loss ; in the second class there is a defect in the perception of colour only. Edridge-Green explains both by an analogy to sound. The first class represents those who are unable to hear very high or very low notes ; the second class represents those who have what may be called a defective musical ear. Both defects may appear in the same individual. The defect in light perception results in a shortened spectrum either at the

---

[1] Sherrington, *Physiological Abstracts*, Vol. 5, p. 161.

red or the violet end—the defect in colour perception causes a less number of colours to be seen than in normal vision.

In this theory colour-blindness is not due to a loss of colour but is caused by the inability of the individuals to detect differences between colours.

CHAPTER III

DESCRIPTION OF TESTS AND DISCUSSION OF RESULTS

1. *Stilling's Pseudo-Isochromatic Tables*

The twelfth edition of the Tables was used. This was generally the first test employed, as it was the first test by means of which the colour-blinds were detected. In conducting experiments with colour with a large body of students it was found that certain students experienced considerable difficulty in carrying out the required experiments owing to a decided inability to detect certain colours. These students were examined in the course of the ordinary laboratory period by means of Stilling's Tables, and some of them failed completely to pass the tests. This led to a more thorough investigation of such cases.

The Tables consist of coloured numbers on a coloured background and there are fourteen in all. Table 1, for example, consists of red numbers on a green ground which are easily distinguishable to the normal eye, but which present great difficulty to certain colour-blinds because there is no contrast effect between the numbers and the background. The Tables are based on the fact that if two colours of equal brightness lie on the same side of the neutral band of the spectrum of the dichromate, they cannot be distinguished.

The Tables test both red-green blindness and blue-yellow blindness, and further differentiate between shortened and unshortened spectrum. Red-green blinds

with normal length of spectrum are unable to read
Tables 1 and 2, but can read Tables 3 and 12 ; red-green
blinds with shortened spectrum *read* Tables 1 and 2,
then 11 and 12, but no others. They have special
difficulty with Table 3. Tables 5, 6, 11 and 12 test
blue-yellow blindness in the same way. Tables 13 and
14 are to detect simulation and every colour-blind is
able to see the figures thereon. The subjects were
tested with all fourteen Tables.

The following are the results obtained :

+ indicates complete pass of the Table.
—   ,,   ,,   failure   ,,
½   ,,   partial success.

	1	2	3	4	5	6	7	8	9	10	11	12	13	14
A	+	+	—	—	—	—	½	—	½	—	½	+	+	+
B	—	—	+	—	—	—	½	—	+	—	½	+	+	+
C	½	½	+	½	½	—	½	—	+	—	½	+	+	+
D	½	½	+	½	½	½	½	½	—	½	—	½	+	+
E	—	—	+	—	—	—	½	—	½	—	+	+	+	+
F	—	—	—	—	—	—	—	—	—	—	½	½	+	+
G	—	—	+	—	—	—	½	—	½	—	½	+	+	+
H	+	+	—	—	—	—	½	—	½	—	½	+	+	+
I	+	+	—	—	—	—	½	—	—	—	+	+	+	+
J	—	—	—	—	—	—	½	—	—	—	½	½	+	+

The Stilling Tables divide the subjects into two
fairly well-marked groups. Five subjects are totally
unable to read Tables 1 and 2 ; two attempt to decipher
the figures with varied success, making many mistakes
but managing a figure here and there. The other three
subjects read the Tables with ease. With Table 3 the
position is reversed. Those unable to read the first two
Tables are delighted to be able to read the third Table
without any difficulty, whereas those who can read easily
the first two Tables find the deciphering of the numbers
in the third Table to be impossible. On a first finding,
then, all subjects are red-green colour-blind. Five of

them have a spectrum shortened at the red end and five of them have a normal length of spectrum. The two subjects who partially pass the Tables show conflicting results in some of the later tests.

One of the subjects discovered that he could read Tables 1 and 2 which before were undecipherable to him, with the aid of a red glass. The red appeared whitish and the green very dark—the contrast between the figures and the background standing out clearly. The subject remarked that he was now convinced that the figures did actually exist, of which he had been sceptical before. Others of the Tables he could read by means of a green glass. In all cases it was merely necessary to obtain a good contrast effect—the red and green glasses absorbed part of the rays of light and neutralized the colours. Red and green glasses have been tried frequently to see if they would cause any palliation of the defect, but they do not seem to have met with much success.

2. Holmgren's Wool Test

The wool test is based on *comparison* of different colours. It was originally suggested by Seebeck and later used by Wilson—of course, in a more or less primitive form. Both investigators recognized that merely testing a colour-blind by naming colours alone was a very inefficient method. Seebeck used about 200 pieces of coloured paper and asked his colour-blinds to sort them. Wilson used skeins of wools in a similar fashion. Holmgren, however, was the first to systematize the test and put it on a scientific basis. He was a staunch adherent of the Young-Helmholtz theory, and, in fact, devised his test in support of the theory.

The wool test has been generally recommended because it has many advantages, such as portability, absence of need for names of colours, and because the wools reflect the light equally in every direction.

The " confusion " skeins, which number over 100, are spread out in irregular order before the subject. They include all varieties of colours and many shades and tints. The examinee is asked to pick out all the skeins the same colour as a given test skein, irrespective of shade. He is told that no two specimens are alike, and that resemblance of colour only is all that is desired.

Holmgren advocates the use of three such test skeins, and those he chose are in agreement with the theory he favoured : a very pale green, a light purple or pink and a full red. The first skein determines the presence of the defect, the second decides if the defect be one of red-blindness or green-blindness, judged by the confusion skeins chosen, the third skein acts as a confirmatory skein.

The tests employed as test skeins in these experiments were not those advocated by Holmgren, but were more or less experimental in character. In all, nine skeins were employed as tests.

1 Vivid green.
2 Vivid red.
3 Brown.
4 Magenta.
5 Green—of medium saturation.
6 Pink—of medium saturation.
7 Very pale green.
8 Very pale pink.
9 Pale blue.

The vivid red, medium pink and pale pink formed a series in intensity which was found to give rather interesting results ; the vivid green, medium green and light green formed a corresponding series in green. These different degrees of intensity of colour were added as the experiment was proceeded with. The magenta was suggested from a reading of Sanford,[1] and the brown suggested from a reading of Abney.[2] The pale blue was added because of a tendency noted to confuse blue and pink, and to ascertain whether the confusion was habitual or merely accidental, and whether it was characteristic of all subjects.

It will be found that the results obtained from testing with the wools seem to point to varying degrees of colour defect.

It is interesting further to note the method employed by the colour-blinds. Their general attitude to the test is important, and the fact as to whether they select their colours with ease or with a great deal of hesitancy. The colour-blinds are very particular with their matches and select the skeins with extreme care. The skeins which they reject are as illuminative of their defect as those they accept and the numbers of both were noted.

We are accustomed to speak of red-green colour-blindness and to mean that the individual cannot distinguish reds or, it may be, greens or both. If he can see red or green then he is no longer colour-blind, but is referred to as colour-weak or as belonging to the class of " anomalous trichromates." We have seen that Professor Hayes challenges that finding, and states that individuals in whose colour system red and green are totally invisible, and blue and yellow the only two colours recognizable,

---

[1] *Experimental Psychology.*
[2] *Researches in Colour-Vision.*

belong to the extreme or limiting class, and that in the typical cases of colour-blindness some kind of red or green is seen by the individual, but not to an extent which would justify his inclusion in the class of anomalous trichromates.

The ten cases examined cannot be classified as cases of colour-weakness showing slight deviation from normality. They all seem to be cases of colour-blindness, but they range from extreme cases in which neither red nor green can be distinguished to cases in which red and green *can* be distinguished with varying degrees of accuracy, if of sufficient intensity. This result is well indicated with Holmgren's wools, and later in the other tests. Fewer mistakes occur with the vivid red and the vivid green than with the pale pink and the pale green—but the number of mistakes varies, of course, according to the extent of the defect.

Results of Wool Test

The results of each skein are separated in order to show the gradual increase in the number of the confusion colours as the defect increases in degree. The subjects are named from A to J, approximately in the order of their deficiency—no rigid series of gradation is intended.

1. *Vivid Green*

A selects greens and brownish greens	rejects olive and green
B ,, ,, ,, ,,	,, olive and brown
C ,, ,, ,, ,,	,, orange, pale blue and brown
D adds yellowish greens	——
E selects greens of all shades and one brown	,, salmon, pink and olive
F selects greens of all shades and yellow, orange, drab	——
G ,, greens and pale brown	——

H selects greens   rejects fawn
I adds, in addition to greens and browns,
          fawns, creams, and yellow,
          orange and salmon   „   pale green
J select sgreens, blue-greens, salmon,
          orange, fawns, reds and
          crimsons, pinks, magenta and
          drabs   „   2 dark greens, 2
                                                   drabs

Subjects A to D match the test skein correctly, which
seems to indicate an ability to select the proper colours.
H also gave correct matches—but he called the test
skein " orange " and selected his matches more for their
brightness than hue. F, G, I and J show confusion—
particularly subject J, who may be regarded as a limiting
case of dichromasy. This subject found it difficult to
imagine what skeins would be like several tones lighter.
It is characteristic of him that he matches each skein
with practically all the confusion skeins—in this case
he had 46 matches.

2. *Vivid Red*

A selects reds and crimsons   ——
B   ,,   reds   rejects a brownish red
C   ,,   reds, crimsons, pink, cinnamons   „   crimson, brown,
                                                pink (too green)
D   ,,   ditto and dark mauve   ——
E   ,,   ditto and light bluish red   „   bluish pink (because
                                                violet)
F   ,,   1 very vivid red, 1 very dark green ——
G   ,,   reds, crimsons, pinks, blues,   „   pale green myrtle,
         purples, drabs and grey   terracotta
H   „   very dark red, greens, pale   ——
         brown
I   „   1 red, different shades of green, „   very dark green and
         brown, blue   very dark crimson
J   „   crimsons, reds, salmon, brown,   ——
         yellows, straws, all shades of
         green, including blue-greens,
         1 pale blue, very dark violet,
         dark slate, drabs

G

A and B select correct matches, which seems to indicate an ability to distinguish red. ⸲The others show the confusion gradually increasing until subject J is reached, and it will be noticed he includes a large assortment of all kinds numbering 52 in all. It seems clear even from these two examples that the defect differs in degree with subjects A and J.

3. *Medium Green*

A	selects	greens and brownish yellow (*N.B.*—confusion beginning)	rejects light orange, canary
B	,,	greens, yellows, orange, brownish yellows and fawns	,, salmon, brown, greenish yellow
C	,,	greens, yellows, orange, brownish yellows and fawns	,, terracotta and a green
D	,,	greens, yellowish greens, and brownish greens	——
E	,,	yellowish and olive greens, fawn, creams, straws, cinnamon, terracotta, salmon	——
F	,,	an emerald and a yellowish green, orange, canary, yellow	,, pale green (because too red), and olive green
G	,,	greens (all shades), yellow, orange, browns and greys, a dark blue and a dark violet	——
H	,,	same as B and C	——
I	,,	greens, cream, yellow, brown	——
J	,,	all shades of green, including blue-greens and brownish greens, browns, reds, very dark slate (almost black), one light orange	,, 1 blue pink, 1 pink, 1 dark mauve

There is a suggestion of the confusion beginning with subject A. She rejects a light orange and a canary. In other words she considered these likely to be matches to a green. B likewise rejects a salmon pink, but he selects as correct yellow and orange skeins. The others show the same confusion as before in increasing measure.

4. *Medium Pink*

A selects pinks, bluish pinks and bluish reds rejects bluish pink
B   „   pinks, bluish pinks and bluish reds   ——
C adds to above pale greens   „   blue, pink and a
                                                        cream
D selects pinks, bluish pinks and bluish reds   „   yellowish fawn
E   „   bluish pinks, yellows, straws,   ——
            creams
F   „   pinks, bluish pinks, violet, pale   ——
            blues, 1 greenish blue, 1 greenish
            grey
. G „   pinks, greens, reds and violets   „   a yellowish fawn
H   „   no pinks, but pale greens, bluish   „   a bluish pink and
            greens, yellowish greens and a   an emerald green
            dark violet
I   „   bluish pinks, blues and greys   ——
J   „   pinks, 1 bluish pink, terracottas,   ——
        . reds and crimsons, greens (all
            shades), greenish greys, greys,
            drabs, straws, browns, blues
            (1 very dark slate blue, 2 royal
            blues, 1 pale blue), 1 dull
            heliotrope

No confusion seems to be existent in cases A, B, D, but
is much in evidence in the other cases. The confusion
between pink and green begins with subject C onwards.
With the vivid red it did not appear until subject F was
reached. Subject J had sixty-seven matches.

5. *Pale Green*

A selects yellows, creams and salmon pink   ——
    (*N.B.*—First confusion of pink and green)
B   „   ditto and pink and orange   rejects greenish yellow
C   „   cream, canary and yellow   „   salmon
D   „   cream, canary and yellow   ——
E   „   different shades of green, yellows, ——
            creams, straws, pinks, salmons,
            pale blues
F   „   same as C   ——
G   „   greens, browns, pinks, greys,   ——
            drab, blues and violets
H   „   same as C   ——
I   „   yellows, pinks, greens, creams   ——
            and orange
J   „   emerald green, cream, canary,   ——
            yellow, orange, fawn

6. *Pale Pink*

A selects bluish pink, yellow-greens, pale   rejects bluish pink
          blues and violets

B   ,,   yellows, pinks, creams, yellow-   ,,   red
          greens and greens

C   ,,   pinks, bluish pink and green   ——

D   ,,   no match   ,,   pale pink and drab

E   ,,   pinks, bluish pinks, greys, straws,   ——
          yellow-greens, pale blue

F   ,,   bluish pinks, blues, pale green   ,,   pink, green, blue
          and greys

G   ,,   no match (skein = dirty white)   ,,   bluish pink and
                                                          emerald green

H   ,,   bluish pinks, pale greens, blues   ,,   pale pink (because
          and greenish blues   too blue)

I   ,,   bluish pinks, vivid blues, reds   ——
          and greys

J   ,,   pinks, 1 blue pink, terracotta,   ——
          reds and crimsons, greens (all
          shades), greenish greys, greys,
          drabs, straws, browns, blue and
          dull heliotrope

With E, F, G, H, I, J, the confusion between red and green is present from the beginning ; with A, red is not confused with green until the very palest skein is to be matched, then the pale green is confused with pink, and there is the usual confusion with yellow. With subject B the confusion is noticeable in the medium green, though not to any great extent, and the confusion increases throughout with more or less regularity. This seems to indicate different degrees of colour defect, which seems to be verified in the later experiments.

7. The *Magenta* skein gave some rather curious results :

A selects reds, bluish pinks, rose pinks,   rejects pink
          pale pinks

B   ,,   blues and violets of all shades,   ,,   vivid blue, violet
          1 bluish red (but not confident   and pink
          about it).

C   ,,   reds and bluish pinks   ,,   lavender, grey,
                                                  violet

D   ,,   crimsons and reds, bluish pinks,   ——
          dark mauve

E selects bluish pinks, rose pinks, violets, ——
   blues
F ,, 1 bluish red, 1 bluish pink, pinks, ——
   very dark purples, violets and
   blues
G ,, crimsons, reds, pinks, bluish reds rejects green, pink, pale
   and mauve   blue
H ,, dark mauve, dark violet, dark ——
   blue and violet
I ,, bluish pink, salmon pink, dark ——
   purple, violets, blues, browns,
   greys, greens, yellow-greens
J ,, magenta reds and medium pinks, ——
   bluish pinks, violets, blues,
   blue greens

B and H matched the test skein with blues and violets
of all shades, and B added one bluish red, evidently
chosen for its bluish element only, although he evinced
considerable hesitation before finally accepting it. When
asked the colour of the skein, both confidently declared
it to be blue. The majority of the others also matched
it with blue and violet, but added some reds as well. I
and J also thought the skein was blue, but their matches
showed considerable confusion. J rejected six skeins,
then accepted them, to reject them later. All were of
bluish or purple shades.

8. The *Brown* skein seemed to cause considerable difficulty.

A Calling the skein dark green, matched it carefully with one skein of
   a very dark olive-green and rejected a green and a brown.
B Matched it with dark greens and brownish greens but rejected all
   pure browns.
C Matched it carefully with two skeins, a very dark crimson and an
   emerald green.
D Matched it with brown, though limited to three in number.
E Matched it with brown and greens.
F Experienced great difficulty in getting any match and finally
   accepted one reddish brown
G *and* I both thought they had been given skein No. 2 again in
   mistake (the vivid red), and expostulated that they had matched
   the brown skein before ! They, therefore, gave similar matches
   as with the former skein, brown, brownish greens, reds and
   crimsons.

H Matched it with greens of all kinds and a few browns.

J As before showed the greatest confusion of all. Crimson, reds, salmon, cinnamon, pure brown, canary, yellow, straws, yellow-greens, greens all shades, blue-green, one pale blue, drabs, very dark violet, dark slate. He rejected 2 dark greens, 2 dark blue-greens, 2 drabs.

It will be noticed that all show confusion, though the confusion seems to increase with the various subjects. Subject J included in his match a pale blue. He thought the skein was a grey and the pale blue a lighter shade of grey. This would seem to indicate a blindness to blue as well, but the subject in some of the tests was found to recognize blue quite easily ; he seems, however, from the evidence to have a weakened sensitivity to blue as well as complete blindness to green and red.

9. The *Blue* skein gave varied results.

A	matched it with	pale blues and greens—no pinks, and thought the skein itself was a pale green	rejects	very pale green, pinks, bluish pinks
B	selects	blues, violets, greens and a bluish pink	,,	bluish pink
C	,,	blues, violets, greens and a bluish pink	,,	pale green, rose
D	,,	blues, pale greens, yellowish greens	,,	pale blue
E	,,	blues, violets, blue-greens, pale greens and greys	——	
F	,,	blues, bluish pink, pinks and a natural grey	,,	blue (because pink)
G	,,	blues, pinks, bluish pinks and crimsons	,,	pale green
H	,,	blues	——	
I	,,	blues, purples, pinks, greens, greys	——	
J	,,	4 blues, 2 very dark slate blues, violets, 26 greens (all shades including blue-, brown-, yellow-greens), pinks, terracotta, reds and crimson, 1 bluish pink, 1 bluish red, 1 very dark red (almost a brown) greys, drabs, straws, canary, brown	——	

The confusion between blue and violet is well marked, which is characteristic of all colour-blinds. There is a confusion also of blue and green. B, C, and D thought the skein was green. The confusion between blue and pink is clearly shown with certain subjects, but is seen not to be characteristic of all subjects. A curious confusion of the skein with grey is common to subjects E, I, J. E called the skein a light blue grey. I said it was either blue or white. J called it a light grey and thought it was the same skein as the pale pink and the medium pink, which he also thought were grey.

The wool test, therefore, gave a considerable insight into the nature of the respective defects of the examinees. All matched the colours very slowly and very deliberately, and often picked up skeins, laid them tentatively beside the others, accepted them, then later rejected them, perhaps to accept them later still. With some the difficulty lay in deciding what the test skein was, and it was turned over and over and viewed at various angles before its colour was finally decided.

If we can assume that the vivid red skein is that similar to the full red of Holmgren, then it does not seem at all a satisfactory colour for a test skein. All subjects did not blunder in matching it, and if used alone it would very often fail to detect colour-blindness. Abney seems to have recognized this fact, for he states that the red skein is the weakest of the three test skeins, and admits that as a test of colour-blindness it is not too satisfactory. It is for this reason that he recommends that a dark brown skein be substituted. A dark brown skein does appear to give a better result and all the subjects found it a difficult colour to match, for brown is one of their most puzzling colours. It does not follow, however, from the results obtained, that the subjects can be divided into two groups according to the confusion colours chosen. Abney states that the red-blind will match not only dark green, but also light green with it ; the green-blind will pick out the browns and the reds. On such a basis subject C would be difficult to place, as he matched it with a very dark crimson and an emerald green ! G, I, J likewise.

The same criticism applies to the other two test skeins as recommended by Holmgren.

The pale-green test is most satisfactory, for it seems to show up the defect immediately. For this reason, too, the pale-pink is most useful. The weaker cases of colour-blindness, as we have seen, are able to pass the test when the colours are more highly saturated. It is the pale colours they have greater difficulty with. Edridge-Green objects to such a green being used as a test skein, and declares it to be the worst possible colour to choose, for the colour-blinds can easily pass through such a test without detection. The results of these experiments do not seem to justify such a conclusion, for all subjects substantially failed in their matches with the pale-green. The medium pinks and greens and the full reds and greens are useful in giving an approximate insight into the extent of the defect, but as tests alone are unreliable.

The magenta skein is also a useful one. All but one subject thought it was blue, or violet, as some called it, and it was astounding to have all shades of blues and violets picked out as good matches. This, too, by subject B, who acquitted himself so well in matching the vivid red skein. It would seem that the blue had been much more powerful than the red to him, and that the red sensation in consequence had suffered. Subject A, on the other hand, gave a good match, although she thought the skein was a purple one. The results, therefore, in her case might be misleading. She has a general confusion of blue and pink, and it would seem that the result she did obtain was due largely to chance. This does not alter the fact, however, that red is visible to her under certain circumstances ; where she confuses blue and pink, or, in this case, magenta and purple, the blue element must be the stronger one, so strong, in fact, that it seems almost to blot out the red sensation.

With the blue skein A made no confusion with blues and pinks in the actual choice she made, but it is noteworthy that she examined one or two pinks and then rejected them ; the confusion was certainly present.

Confusion of blue with pink is said to be characteristic of a shortened spectrum. If the pink is made up of a mixture of red and violet, the red element is invisible, and the violet remains, which is seen as blue. Subject G, however, who has no shortening of the spectrum—if Stilling's Tables are trustworthy—also shows a similar confusion.

In conducting this wool test, Holmgren advises that the examiner, in cases where a verbal explanation fails, should resort to actually showing the individual how the selection should be done, and he argues that " no one with a defective chromatic sense finds the correct skeins in the pile the more easily from the fact of having a moment before seen others looking for and arranging them."[1] From practical experience in testing colour-blinds, this method must be strongly deprecated. A shrewd colour-blind, once he obtains a clue to the colours required, will make a wonderful show of accuracy. Further, Holmgren's second instruction, that in testing large numbers the candidate should be instructed " to attentively observe

[1] Jeffries : *Colour-Blindness : Its Dangers and its Detection*, p. 211. Translation from Holmgren.

the examination of those preceding them," seems to be defeating the purpose of the test.

ᶠ The great advantage of Holmgren's test is that it is based on comparing colours, not on naming colours. Certainly, when Holmgren devised his test, it was a step in the right direction, for the testing of colour-blinds by naming alone is most unsatisfactory. But in conducting the wool test just described, the subject was always asked what colour he thought the test skein was, and his answers were most illuminating, and increased the value of the test tenfold. The author has since discovered that Edridge-Green in his classification test, which is a modified wool test employing different test skeins, advocates the same procedure. In fact, the candidate is asked to name each colour as he selects it. It was found most instructive, too, to ask the names of the rejected colours, and why they were rejected, and the reasons throw considerable light upon the colour defect. The combined method, therefore, of comparing and naming seems to yield the best results.

In conclusion, the most outstanding result of this series of tests is the confirmation of Professor Hayes' results, that there are varying degrees of red-green colour-blindness. The graded series of reds and greens brought this result clearly out, and it will be found that later experiments point strongly in the same direction.

3. *Colour Naming*

Tests involving colour naming have come in for a large share of hostile criticism, and were considered as unsatisfactory by the Committee appointed to report on Colour-Vision, in 1892. " Tests which involve the naming of colours should be avoided in deciding the question of colour-blindness."[1] The colour-blinds judge of colours by differences in shade, and a difference in shade to them often means a difference in colour. They hear a colour called red which to them may appear as a very dark yellow and they associate the name and the shade together. In some cases their skill in using correct colour names is remarkable, and renders the detection of their defect more difficult.

Dr Pole himself remained ignorant of his defect for thirty years. Dalton, too, in speaking of some of his pupils, remarked, " They, like all the rest of us colour-blinds, were not aware of their actually seeing colours different from other people, but imagined there was great perplexity in the *names* ascribed to particular colours."

It was for this reason that Holmgren devised his test, which obviates the need for colour names. " To judge correctly of colour-blindness, and the various practical questions connected with it, it is of the highest importance to distinctly observe the difference between the manner in which the colour-blind *sees*, and the manner in which he *names*, colours. The sensation is based upon the nature of the sense of colours in the organization of the optic nerve from birth. The *name*, on the contrary, is learned. It is conventional ; it depends upon exercise and habit. The names of colours are naturally the objective expression of subjective sensations ; but, on the other hand, they are regulated by the system of normal sight, and cannot consequently agree with that of the colour-blind."[2]

The objection which Holmgren had against testing by naming colours seems to have arisen from the fact that such a test used to be applied to detect colour-blinds in

[1] *Proceedings of the Royal Society of London*, Vol. 51.
[2] Quoted from Jeffries, *Colour-Blindness: Its Dangers and its Detection*, p. 94.

a most haphazard manner, and no other test was added. Colour naming is a useful test, but it must be of a supplementary nature. Alone, it is most unreliable, particularly if names of familiar objects are asked for.

Dr Jeffries, to test this point, conducted an interesting questionnaire with blind children—children blind from birth to form as well as to colour. He asked them the colours of familiar objects such as the sky, an apple, banana, strawberry, grass, leaves, water, etc., and received curious answers. For example, to banana, he received the following replies: "Don't know," "No idea," "Yellow," "Don't know," "Don't know," "Green— uncertain." These were children ranging in age from ten to nineteen. Unfortunately, the experiment could not be continued, for colours became the topic of conversation throughout the institution after that. The colours of grass and cherry, however, were fairly well known. "Through the ear alone these answers were learned, and retained by memory. The attachment of the name of a colour to an object is an attribute not learned by the eye alone. A wholly uneducated person who handles bricks if he hears them called black will so call them when questioned as to their colour."[1] This is a similar condition to that found in the colour-blind. He learns by the ear the names and colours of familiar objects. He associates the colour name in some cases with the eye sensation which he experiences on seeing the object which may be some finely discriminated shade. In consequence, he is often able to give correctly a colour name, although he does not actually see that particular colour.

Edridge-Green, however, adopts an entirely different attitude, and is a strong advocate in favour of testing nomenclature, particularly for practical purposes. He introduces colour naming into his classification test and

[1] Jeffries, *Colour-Blindness: Its Dangers and its Detection*, p. 100.

into his lantern test. The latter test, in its relation to colour naming, we shall consider later. As long as the objects to be named are carefully chosen, colour naming gives considerable insight into the colour-blind's defect. It will be found that in many cases the colour-blind does not guess the names of colours ; he has a regular system of his own to which he firmly adheres.

To test the validity of colour naming two methods were tried :

1 The naming of the dots in Stilling's Tables.

2 The naming of Holmgren's wools.

Some of the subjects were tested after the lapse of a year, and their colour nomenclature was found to remain constant. This confirms the view that guessing is not the rule, but that the colour-blinds are guided by definite colour sensations which give them a regular colour system.

(a) Stilling's Tables

Table 1

Red (light and medium) figures on *Green* (light and medium) background

A	red	green
B	red	green
C	dark green and brown	yellow and brown
D	red	dark green
E	violet	grey
F	red ?	yellow and green
G	red	green
H	brown	yellow and orange
I	green and red	green or yellow and green
J	All shades of grey	

The colour names employed are characteristic of the defect, and it must be admitted they reveal how great that defect is. Subject B, though recognizing the colours, could not decipher the figures. Subject C could partially read the figures, although it will be noticed that his nomenclature shows considerable confusion. This is characteristic of him throughout all the tests. Being questioned, he declared he had no interest in colours at all, and had not thought whether he confused them or not. Finally, he admitted that crimsons and the finer shades were difficult for him, but the question of colour in general seemed to have caused him no concern. J, as before, shows the defect to be much graver than the others, and sees all colours as shades of grey.

Table 2

Green (light and medium) figures on *Red* (light and dark) background
(light dots resembling a fawn colour)

A	green	red
B	orange red and red	red
C	yellow and dark green	light green and dark red
D	dark green	light and dark brown
E	bright green	greyish green and grey
F	yellow and　?	green and red
G	yellow and green	red and green
H	yellow and orange	dark brown and black
I	green	red and black
J	different shades of grey	

How does this compare with the first Table? A's results are similar to those in the first Table—she recognizes red and green. B, however, shows confusion this time. Yellow is evidently confused with pale-green in the cases of subjects C, F and H—a common confusion. J remains constant, and sees all as shades of grey. One other point of interest worth noting is in the case of subject H— the medium green which resembles somewhat a grass green, he calls orange. This is characteristic of him, and tested a year later the same naming held good. This is verified in the other tests. Note also that he calls the red black—this at once indicates a shortened spectrum.

Table 3

Bright Red figures on *Mole and Black* background

A	red	green
B	red	green and black
C	red	green
D	dark red	brown
E	red	green
F	light red	darker shades of red
G	red	green and dark green
H	brown	grey and black
I	grey	shades of grey
J	black	shades of grey

The red used in this Table is a very bright red, and was recognized as such by subjects A to G. This particular shade of red, which seems similar to that used in the Nagel cards, gave similar results there. It will be noticed that the background contains a difficult colour for them, one of these indefinite colours which is always a puzzle for them, and which rarely fails to detect them. The majority have called it green. J, as before, sees all the colours as grey—red is seen as black, which denotes a shortened spectrum. Subject H sees this shade of red as brown—that is, a dark shade of red is black, a medium shade is brown for this subject.

Table 4

Red figures on *Fawn and Mole* background

A	red	green and black
B	red	green
C	red	dark green
D	red	dark brown
E	red	dark green and grey
F	red	green
G	red	green
H	grey and black	grey and brown
I	grey	brown and black
J	black	shades of grey

Red again is recognized by subjects A to G. It is of the same particular brightness as in Table 3. H and J confirm

the shortened spectrum. The background contains confusion colours which are not recognized.

Table 5

Fawn and Red figures on *Grey and Mole* background

A	green and red	green
B	shades of green	green
C	green	green
D	shades of brown	dark brown
E	grey and red	grey
F	light red	red
G	green	green
H	grey and brown	grey
I	grey	brown and green
J	different shades of grey	

The red in this Table is a dull red—what might be called
a "blae" colour—and few subjects could identify it. This
is a striking difference from the last Table. It seems to
point to the fact that the colour must be somewhat
resembling what may be designated as a " pure red "
in order that it may be identified. It must be reds
like these which are confused with greens. The background, as before, shows grey mistaken for green.
Note subject J again—he truly seems a limiting case of
dichromasy.

Table 6

Fawn and Red figures on *Grey and Mole* background (dots,
however, larger in size)

A	red	green
B	crimson	green
C	green or brown	green
D	shades of brown	dark grey
E	all different shades of grey	
F	light red	dark red
G	red and green	green
H	grey and brown	grey and light brown
I	dark grey	green
J	different shades of grey	

A and B this time recognize the red, but otherwise the naming remains very similar to the preceding Table, except with E, who sees the colours as shades of grey.

Table 7

Crimson figures on *Brown and Brownish-green* background

A	red	green
B	crimson	green
C	brown	brown
D	red	grey
E	dark brown	brown and dark green
F	red	?
G	red	brown
H	brown and black	two shades of brown
I	dark brown and black	dark grey
J	different shades of grey	

This confirms the previous Tables, that red under certain circumstances can be recognized. The background shows confusion of green and brown. Subject I now shows signs of a shortened spectrum, because of confusion of red and black. That is from colour naming alone, H, I and J have been found to have shortened spectrum, which verifies the results obtained from the reading of the Tables.

Table 8

Bright Red and Crimson figures on *Brown and Greenish-brown* background

A	red	green
B	crimson	red and green
C	brown	light brown
D	dark red	brown
E	red	dark green
F	red	brown
G	red	green
H	brown	brown and grey
I	dark grey or black	shades of brown
J	different shades of grey	

H

The red here is fairly well recognized because it is of this bright variety. Subject C, however, calls it brown. His nomenclature is not good throughout, and shows considerable confusion. This is curious when we remember that he can partially pass the Stilling Tables so far as deciphering the numbers is concerned.

Table 9

Pink figures on *Brown and Dark Brown* background

A	red	green and red
B	greenish red	brown and black
C	green	brown
D	dark brown	grey
E	medium grey	brown
F	light red	?
G	green	green
H	black	grey and black
I	green and brown	brown or red
J	figures decidedly lighter ; all, however, shades of grey	

This Table gives interesting results—all show confusion. Note the description given by B of the figures, greenish red. This term is characteristic of the mild forms of colour-blindness and of cases, too, where red seems sometimes to be recognized. No two call both colours the same. J still maintains his different shades of grey. Evidently he has not learned to associate a shade with the name of a colour. Subject E has more than once called a colour a grey, and it was he who called the blue skein in the Holmgren's wools a grey. Does this suggest a lowered sensitivity to colours in general? Subject F is very often completely at a loss as to the name of a colour, and finds it impossible to make even a guess at it. It will also be noticed that green is more often mentioned than red, which shows, we may tentatively suggest, that, when in doubt, green is the accepted solution.

Table 10.

Red figures on *Fawn and Brown* background

A	red	green and red
B	red	green and reddish brown
C	red	green and brown
D	all dark red	shades of grey
E	red	light green
F	red	may be brown
G	red and green	nondescript and green
H	brown	grey and brown
I	brown	green
J	different shades of grey	

Brown and red are often mistaken for one another ; further, as we have already noticed, green and fawn are liable to be confused. The red is more correctly and more frequently distinguished than the green and does not seem liable to the same amount of confusion. Often the background which contains two shades of the same colour is described as red and green—a difference in shade means a difference in colour.

Table 11

Crimson figures on *Orange and Brown* background

A	red	green and red
B	crimson	orange and green
C	red	yellow
D	red	red and grey
E	red	light brown
F	red	yellowish tinge
G	red	yellow and red
H	black	orange and brown
I	dark grey	light brown or green and dark brown
J	figures are black against the background	

The red figures are well recognized again, except for the last three subjects, who are well-marked cases of shortened spectrum, and who in consequence see the red as black. The orange and brown both proved difficult colours. Note that subject A confuses brown and red, therefore red cannot always be a clear sensation for her.

Table 12

Yellow-green (light and dark) figures on *Blue* (light and dark)
background

A	yellow-green and green	blue
B	shades of green	different shades of blue
C	green and brown	green and blue
D	shades of green	very light grey and dark blue
E	green and light brown	slate colour
F	colours vary (no idea)	red and dark blue
G	green	blue
H	shades of grey	grey and blue
I	green and brown	pink and blue
J	white	medium grey and blue (hesitation)

Two things are of interest here :

(1) The light shade of blue is often seen as pale grey.
This confirms the results obtained in matching the wools,
and seems to be characteristic of some colour-blinds. J
was doubtful about the blue, and finally described it as
being the colour of ink.

(2) The light shade of blue is confused with pink. This
is a further sign of a shortened spectrum. F and I, who
show this confusion, have a shortened spectrum, for they
cannot decipher the figures in Table 3.

Table 13

Crimson figures on *Fawn and Mole* background

A	red	two different greens
B	crimson	two different greens
C	brown	green
D	dark red	two greys
E	dark red	light grey
F	darker shade	shades of brown
G	red brown	green
H	black	grey and brown
I	black or dark grey	green and brown
J	black	shades of grey

The last three again show signs of shortened spectrum ;
the others show a discrimination of red. Fawn and mole,
as before, are confused with green. Note F's indefinite
phraseology.

Table 14
  Crimson (light and dark) figures on *Brown and Mole* background

A	red	green
B	crimson red	reddish green
C	brown	light brown
D	light grey and dark grey	very light grey and brown
E	dark brown	green
F	may be dark red	darker shades
G	brown and ?	green
H	black	all brown
I	dark grey or brown	light brown
J	black	fairly dark grey

This particular red is not so well recognized. The last three, as before, call it black. Subject B employs his former terminology and designates the background as reddish green. C and D, who partially pass the Stilling's tests so far as reading the numbers is concerned, are bad at colour naming. This Table shows clearly the confusions they make. Further, the background, as before, shows how greatly green is confused with brown. The puzzling colours seem more liable to be called green than to be called red.

From the results of colour naming, various facts may be deduced.

(1) There are different grades of colour-blindness ranging from extreme cases in which no red and green can be perceived to cases in which red and green can be perceived under certain circumstances. Subject J is the extreme case.

(2) Red, if of sufficient brightness, can be distinguished by some colour-blinds. (*Vide* subjects A and B.)

(3) Red is seen as black by those with shortened spectrum.

(4) Red is confused with blue in certain cases of shortened spectrum.

(5) Brown is a common confusion colour of green.

(6) Greenish red is a colour name employed by colour-blinds.

(7) Pale blue in some cases of red-green blindness is seen as pale grey.

(8) Partial passing of the Tables does not coincide with good nomenclature.

(9) Finally, and this is perhaps the most important result obtained, the colour-blinds do not guess names of colours, but have a regular colour system which determines the names they employ.

It will be seen, therefore, that a large amount of information has been gathered from merely asking the examinees to name colours, and that an insight into their respective defects has been obtained.

(Red appears 13 times in the Tables.)

A	recognized it	13	times
B	,,	11	,,
C	,,	4	,,
D	,,	8	,,
E	,,	7	,,
F	,,	9	,,
G	,,	7	,,
H	,,	0	,,
I	,,	0	,,
J	,,	0	,,

The above Table speaks for itself, and shows the great variety among the ten colour-blinds examined. The case of C is a curious one, and all through his results are conflicting. The recognition of red only 4 times would seem to place him much nearer the extreme case, and some experiments would verify this, but others, again, would make his defect appear less grave. Note H, I and J failed completely to identify red.

(b) *The Naming of Holmgren's Wools*

All the skeins were named by each colour-blind. Below are a few samples of the names given. The full list is appended.

Colour of Skein	A	B	C	D	E	F	G	H	I	J
1 vivid green	green	green	red or yellow or brown	green	green	yellow	green	orange	green	light grey
2 vivid red	red	red	red	red	red	red	red	brown	brown	nearly black
3 brown	dark green	green	very dark green	brown	dark brown	brownish tinge	green	brown	brown	dark grey
4 magenta	purple	blue	blue and red	very dark red	violet	reddish blue	pink	blue	blue or purple	dark blue
5 medium green	yellow	green	green	green	light brown	yellow and red	fawn and green	yellow	green	medium grey
6 medium pink	pink	pink	light green	very pale grey	nearly white	red and some other colour	pink	grey	pale blue	light grey
7 light green	yellow or pink	green	yellowish green	green	light brown	red	green	yellow	yellow or blue green	yellow
8 light pink	pink	pink	light green	dark grey	flesh	? might be red	dirty white	greyish white	white or blue	light grey
9 pale blue	pale green	greenish blue	green and blue	light green	blue-grey	blue	blue	blue	white or blue	light grey
10 straw	pink	pale yellow	brown and yellow	cream	cream	white	pink	pink	green	light grey
11 drab	green	grey	green	brown	grey	red	green	dark blue	green	medium grey
12 very dark violet	violet	greenish brown	green	slate	slate	some red in it	slate	slate	pinkish greenish brownish	medium grey
13 rose	pink	pink	green and red about it	pink	pink	red	pink	blue	blue	? blue

These few examples give characteristic results. Very pale greys, drabs and creams are usually thought to be pale pinks or pale greens. Subjects A, B, D, E only confused the pale shades, and subject A volunteered the information that she could distinguish bright shades without difficulty—it was just the pale shades of colours which she knew she confused. Subject C's nomenclature is very bad—in fact, is misleading. In colour mixing he could distinguish differences between colours to a very fine degree, although he would call a pink green and a green red. He is very fond of using the terms greenish red or reddish green—a pink is, in lack of a colour term, described as composed of green and red; similarly lavender is composed of blue and green; a bluish red, a bluish pink and a pale green are all composed of red and green. This verifies the results obtained from the naming of Stilling's Tables.

Subject I's nomenclature is, perhaps, worse, but it coincides with his colour matches. Pinks of all shades he calls blues, reds are called browns, and greens yellow. Orange cannot be distinguished from yellow nor purple or violet from blue—reds and greens change names promiscuously. He was very proud of one colour—a very dark green which he claimed twice over with evident satisfaction to be crimson lake.

A summary of his results runs as follows :—Dark crimson and red he calls brown; pink is blue, sometimes green, orange is yellow; yellow is yellow or green; but the yellow element can always be distinguished in compound colours such as a yellowish green; yellow green is yellow; dark olive green is brown, but twice called crimson lake; emerald green is dark yellow; pale green is grey or pink; blue green is called brown, but if very pale is described as a dirty white; blue is sometimes called blue, sometimes called purple ; pale blue is pink ; violet usually blue, sometimes pink ; brown is called brown, green or red ; all greys, drabs or straws are called greens or pinks.

The other subjects show somewhat similar results with variations here and there.

Subject J, however, sees the colours as a monotonous series of shades of grey. A glance down the column in which his results are recorded shows that yellow and blue are the sole colour names of his vocabulary. Four times he calls dark green brown, and once he ventures the name purple and once the name orange ; but, apart from these instances, yellow and blue are his only colours.

The wools give a more varied result than the Stilling's Tables, simply because there is a larger variety of hues.

We see subject F's indefinite phraseology continued, " some red in it," " red and something else," " might be red," and so on, which characterized his naming in the Tables. We find the same confusion of green, and yellow, and brown, and grey ; of pink and blue ; of red and brown, and red and black ; of violet and blue. Further we find the phrase "reddish green " used with fair frequency.

The results from colour naming, therefore, are not to be despised, for they yield a large return.

HOLMGREN'S WOOLS

Where no colours are given colours were named correctly

l. = light   p. = pale   d. = dark   v. = very   med. = medium

	A	B	C	D	E	F	G	H	I	J
1 Straw	pink	p. yellow	brown and yellow	—	—	white	green	pink	green	l. grey
2 Greenish grey	—	d. grey	green	—	—	green	green	blue	green	med. grey
3 Rose pink	—	—	green with red about it	—	—	red	—	—	blue	? blue
4 Emerald green	—	—	—	—	grey	yellow	—	d. grey	—	med. grey
5 L. orange	—	yellow	yellow	—	yellow	—	—	—	yellow	d. yellow
6 P. green	grey	—	—	—	l. grey	—	—	grey	—	med. grey
7 P. pink	—	—	l. green	l. grey	—	—	—	—	blue	l. grey
8 P. green	—	—	—	—	—	grey white	p. green	yellowish white	—	v. d. grey
9 Canary	—	—	—	—	yellow and brown	—	—	—	—	—
10 P. brown	green	—	—	brown	—	d. brown	greenish brown	—	—	—
11 V. d. purple	blue	blue	d. blue	—	blue	blue	—	—	—	d. blue
12 Blue	—	—	—	—	brown	red	p. red	grey	—	med. grey
13 Cream	pink	—	green and yellow	—	—	white	—	—	—	v. l. yellow
14 Emerald green	—	yellow	—	—	—	yellow	—	orange	d. yellow	d. yellow
15 V. d. red brown	pink	—	l. brown	brown	red	brown	—	d. brown	brown	v. d. grey
16 Salmon pink	—	p. yellow	—	yellow	v. l. brown	green	red	orange	green	med. grey
17 V. p. green	green	p. blue	—	—	l. grey	greyish white	—	grey	blue	l. grey
18 Vivid pink	—	—	—	—	—	reddish blue	—	orange	—	? blue
19 P. yellowish green	brown	p. yellow	blue and green	—	brown	yellowish brown	—	—	—	l. grey
20 Yellowish green	yellow	yellow	yellow	—	—	yellow	yellow	yellow	yellow	d. yellow
21 Cinnamon	—	—	—	—	—	—	salmon	—	greenish brown	med. grey
22 Drab	green	—	green	brown	—	red	red	—	green	med. grey
23 Fawnish yellow	pink	—	—	brown	—	—	salmon	d. blue	pink	yellow
24 V. d. crimson brown	—	—	fawn green and brown	d. grey	d. brown	brown	—	brown	d. brown	black
25 Yellowish fawn	—	—	red	—	—	—	—	—	green	fairly l. grey
26 Red	—	—	—	—	—	green	green	grey	blue	d. grey
27 Fawn	—	—	—	—	—	—	—	grey	green	med. grey
28 Bottle green	—	—	—	—	—	red with brown in it	—	—	—	d. grey

HOLMGREN'S WOOLS—continued

		A	B	C	D	E	F	G	H	I	J
29	Orange	darker yellow	d. yellow	yellow	brown	—	yellow	—	—	yellow	d. yellow
30	Bluish pink	—	—	red and green	red	red	blue	—	blue	blue	purple?
31	Pale cream	pink	—	l. green almost yellow	brown	yellowish brown	white	p. yellow and red	—	green	l. yellow
32	Pea green	—	—	yellow	blue	—	red and white	—	grey	yellow or green	med. grey
33	Yellow	—	—			—		—		blue	
34	P. violet	pink	blue	l. blue	blue	pink	blue	red	blue	l. blue	l. blue
35	P. green	pink	p. yellow	—	blue or green	l. brown	—	—	grey	—	l. grey
36	Pinkish yellow	pink	p. yellow	v. l. green	brown	l. brown	white	p. red	pinkish	green	l. grey
37	Geranium Pink	—	—	—	green	—	—	—	—	purple brown	med. grey
38	D. blue	—	—	—	—	—	—	—	—	—	d. grey
39	D. green, almost black	—	—	—	—	—	green? some red in it	—	d. grey	d. grey	d. grey
40	D. slate blue	green	d. grey	green	—	—	some red in it	d. green	d. grey	—	
41	V. d. violet	—	greenish brown	green	—	—	—	slate	—	pinkish greenish brownish	med. grey
42	Jade green	grey	—	—	—	l. grey	orange	—	grey	yellow-brown	med. grey
43	D. olive green	—	—	brown	—	—	—	—	grey	—	d. grey
44	Dull helio.	—	blue with something else	green	—	—	red	blue green	grey blue	d. pink	bluey grey
45	V. d. blue	—	—	—	—	d. blue, d. grey	—	—	—	—	d. blue
46	P. crimson	pink	—	reddish green brown	—	brown	—	—	brown	brown with pink in it	med. grey
47	Brownish green	—	l. brown	brown	—	brown	d. brown	—	d. orange	golden brown	d. grey
48	Blue pink	—	green and blue in it	green	grey	red in it	blue	—	l. blue	blue	med. grey
49	Grey (nat.)	—	—	l. green	—	—	red	red	pink	pink	l. grey
50	P. bluish pink	—	p. yellow	l. green	grey	flesh	red	—	white	greenish brown	l. grey
51	P. green	—	—	—	—	—	—	—	l. brown	—	l. grey
52	Blue green	—	—	blue and green	—	grey green	red	—	grey	brown with pink in it	med. grey

HOLMGREN'S WOOLS—*continued*

	A	B	C	D	E	F	G	H	I	J
53 Pink	—	—	green and red	—	—	—	—	blue	blue	l. grey
54 Crimson	—	—		—	—	—	—	d. brown	brown	v. d. grey
55 Brownish green		reddish yellow brown	l. brown	—	l. brown	orange	—	orange	golden brown	orange
56 Olive green	brown	brown	green and brown	—		brown	—	brown	—	fairly d. grey
57 P. green	—	yellow	red and green	—	brownish green	some red ?	l. green	orange	d. pink	l. grey
58 Emerald green			brownish yellow	—		yellow	blue green / blue		yellow	d. yellow
59 Grey	greenish	blue	l. green	—	d. steel grey	l. red	—	pink	pink	l. grey
60 V. d. blue green	blue	d. blue	—	blue	green with pink in it	red ?	—	almost grey	crimson lake	v. d. grey
61 P. blue green		blue	blue		—	l. grey	—	white	dirty white	l. grey
62 Pink	—	greenish blue	green	—	—	red	—	brown	blue or pink	med. grey
63 Almost grey slate blue				grey			p. green		greenish bluish	l. grey
64 Royal	—	—	brown	—	brown	d. brown	—	pink	brown	l. blue
65 V. d. olive green	—	d. brown	—	—	l. blue	some red and ?	p. green		dirty white	d. grey
66 Sea green	—	—	—	—		—	—			l. grey
67 Green	—	grey	blue and green / greenish blue	—	grey with green in it	blue	—	d. grey	brown with pink in it	fairly d. grey
68 Lavender	blue	blue	brown	blue	blue ?		—	blue	blue	med. blue
69 Blue	—	—	brown	—	blue grey	brown	blue	brown	brown	d. grey
70 D. olive green	—	brown		—		red	—		brown	med. grey
71 Green	blue		red and green	—	blue grey / red	blue	green	l. blue	blue	touch of blue
72 Bluish pink		p. blue	green	—		red / blue	—		jade green / pinkish	
73 Greenish blue	—	greenish brown		—	blue grey	red and brown	green	—	greenish brownish	l. grey
74 Grey	green			—	brown		—		brownish green	med. grey
75 P. terra-cotta	—	—	—	fawn	brown	green	reddish pink	l. brown	brownish green	fairly d. grey
76 Blue	—	blue	blue	green blue	—	—	blue	—	golden brown	d. blue
77 Violet		brown	l. brown	—	—	—	—	blue	—	grey
78 Emerald green				—		orange	—	orange	golden brown	med. grey

HOLMGREN'S WOOLS—*continued*

		A	B	C	D	E	F	G	H	I	J
79	Myrtle green	d. green	Almost black green	—	—	d. grey	red ? brown	d. green	grey	d. grey	d. grey
80	D. mauve	—	d. brown	blue	—	blue	blue	—	blue	—	d. blue
81	V. d. green	—	blue	—	—	d. grey	red or ? brown	blue	d. grey	crimson lake	black
82	Brownish green	—	—	brown	—	brown	brown	—	brown	brown	d. grey
83	Blue green	—	—	red and green	—	—	red blue	—	—	—	med. blue
84	Bluish red	—	pink	—	—	—	blue	—	—	purple	d. grey
85	P. violet	blue	blue	blue	blue	blue	blue	blue	brown	brown	med. blue
86	Brownish green	—	l. brown	brown	—	brown	brown	brown	—	pink	brown
87	Grey	pink	—	—	yellow	—	red	green	—	yellow and brown	l. grey
88	L. olive green almost blue	—	l. brown	l. brown	—	green and brown	orange	—	orange	dirty white	l. grey
89	P. green	—	greenish	red and green	d. grey	green ?	some red	p. green	pink	purple	l. grey
90	Brown	green	brownish	green and brown	—	—	—	green	blue	—	d. grey
91	Blue	—	blue	blue	—	blue	blue	blue	—	—	—
92	D. violet	—	brown	brown	—	brown	brown	—	—	brown	p. blue
93	D. greenish brown	brown	—	blue green	—	—	—	—	—	pink	brown
94	Sea blue	—	bluish pink	blue and green	—	—	brown	—	—	brown	d. grey
95	Emerald green	—	—	—	brown	—	red	pink	—	pink	l. grey
96	P. blue	p. green	—	green	—	—	—	—	—	—	—
97	Grey green	—	d. grey greenish	d. green	l. green	d. grey	red	pink	—	brown red	brown
98	P. blue	p. green	blue	green and blue	—	l. blue	—	—	—	white or blue	l. grey
99	Terra-cotta	—	—	—	crimson	grey	brown	red	—	brown	d. grey
100	P. blue	—	—	brownish green	—	brown	—	—	—	—	—
101	P. brown	—	brown	—	—	—	green	green	—	—	d. grey
102	Blue	—	—	—	green	blue grey	red brown	—	—	brown or red	—
103	D. green	—	—	—	—	d. grey	—	—	grey	—	d. grey
104	L. violet	—	blue	blue	blue	l. blue	blue	blue	—	blue or purple	l. blue
105	Violet	—	—	—	blue green	—	—	—	blue	—	l. blue
106	Violet	blue	blue	—	—	blue	blue	—	brown	—	l. blue
107	Olive green	brown	l. brown	green	—	l. brown	brown	—	—	pinkish	med. grey
108	P. blue	p. green	—	—	—	—	red	—	—	—	l. grey
109	D. blue	—	—	—	—	grey-blue	reddish blue	—	—	—	—
110	Olive green	—	l. brown	—	—	—	brown	—	brown	—	brown

HOLMGREN'S WOOLS—*continued*

| | | | | | TEST SKEINS | | | | | |
	A	B	C	D	E	F	G	H	I	J
1 Vivid green	—	—	red, yellow, brown	—	green	yellow	—	orange	—	l. grey
2 Vivid red	—	—	red	—	red	red	—	brown	brown	black
3 Brown	d. green	green	v. d. green	—	d. brown	brown tinge	green	brown	brown	fairly d. grey
4 Magenta	purple	blue	blue and red	v. d. red	violet	reddish blue	pink	blue	blue or purple	fairly d. blue
5 Med. green	yellow	—	green	—	l. brown	yellow or red	fawn and green	yellow	—	med. grey yellow tinge
6 Med. pink	—	—	l. green	v. p. grey	nearly white	red and ? white	—	grey	p. blue	l. grey
7 V. p. green	yellow or pink	—	yellowish green	—	l. brown	red	—	yellow	yellow or blue-green	yellow
8 V. p. pink	—	—	l. green	d. grey	flesh	? red	dirty white	grey white	white or p. blue	l. grey
9 V.p. blue	p. green	greenish-blue	green and blue	l. green	l. blue-grey	—	pink	—	white or blue	l. grey

CHAPTER IV

TESTS AND RESULTS—*continued*

4. *Colour Equations*

Colour mixing, to detect colour defect, seems to have originated with Professor Clerk Maxwell, who devised his Colour Top. Since then this method has gained considerable favour in the diagnosis of abnormalities of colour-vision.

In the series of experiments conducted, the Bradley colour papers were employed. These all profess to be pure spectral colours. The discs were rotated in the usual way on an electric colour-wheel.

A circular piece of stout paper with a small hole in the centre is fixed on the colour-wheel. In front of this, a large uncut disc is placed, or two large discs with edges cut along one radius, as the case may be. If there are two discs they are interlocked so that their proportions can be easily adjusted. In front of these large discs, and on the same wheel, smaller discs of paper are fixed. When the wheel is rotated, the colours of the larger discs are thrown so rapidly in succession on the retina that they mix and form one colour. Similarly, the smaller discs appear of one hue. The object of the experiment is to make the colour obtained from the inner discs identical in hue and brightness with the colour obtained from the outer discs when in rotation.

Such a method reveals the great difference which exists between the normal and the colour-defective eye.

Matches are made by the colour-blind which appear absurd to the normal eye ; and reds and greens, in many cases, appearing colourless to them, can be matched with greys. Consequently, equations are obtained which reveal the defect of the colour-blind. As far as possible the intensity of light must be kept constant.

In this series of experiments an equation for green was tried first of all. 360° green was rotated on the wheel and in front of it two smaller interlocked discs of black and white respectively were simultaneously rotated, an endeavour being made to get the outer and the inner discs to match. The black and white discs were adjusted according to the wish of the examinee until he was perfectly satisfied with the match. The proportions were then measured by means of a circular protractor. The colour-blind are very careful in matching colours, and express intense dissatisfaction if the slightest difference is visible. Ten colour equations were tried in all, and each subject was tested with the complete set.

1	Green	=black+white
2	Red	=black+white
3	Red	=green
4	Red	=yellow+black
5	Green+red (+blue)	=black+white
6	Blue+yellow	=black+white
7	*Green	=yellow+black
8	Violet	=blue+black
9	Orange	=yellow+black
10	Orange	=green

Below are the exact Bradley colours employed.

Red	=red tint 1
Green	=blue-green
Yellow	=yellow tint 1
Violet	=violet shade 2
Orange	=orange
Blue	=blue
*Green	=green

(1) *Green = Black + White*

	Green + White			Black + White		
A	360		=	216	+	144
B	360		=	249	+	111
C	—					
D	15	+ 345	=	20	+	340
E	122	+ 238	=	135	+	225
F	86	+ 274	=	34	+	326
G	360		=	241	+	119
H	360		=	193	+	167
I	197	+ 163	=	110	+	250
J	360		=	249	+	111

In this case, five of the subjects were able to obtain a perfect match—others required the green to be diluted with white before seeing it as a grey. The results of these five show a curious correspondence—in fact, the equations of B and J, the two extremes as we may call them, are identical. This would indicate for these particular subjects a complete blindness to green, or rather, blue-green. Later, it was found that the blue-green in the spectrum formed a neutral band for them. For a considerable time H saw pink in the black-white disc where no pink was visible to examiner, whereas the final match, which to H seemed perfect, appeared pinkish to examiner. The other subjects required the green to be diluted with white before it could be matched with a grey. In all cases, however, except in those of subjects C and D, the green was clearly visible to examiner. The equations of C and D were excellent and perfectly normal —C's was not recorded, but it was very similar to that of D. This is curious when their nomenclature is remembered—but it agrees with the fact that they did better than the other subjects in the Stilling Test.

I

(2) *Red = Black + White*

	Red + White			=	Black + White		
A	85	+	275	=	89	+	271
B	82	+	278	=	68	+	292
C	———————				———————		
D	22·5 +		337·5	=	11	+	349
E	49	+	311	= .	64	+	296
F	102	+	258	=	115	+	245
G	143	+	217	=	33	+	327
H	253	+	107	=	229	+	131
I	195	+	165	=	278	+	82
J	360			=	342	+	18

This series of equations clearly shows a difference in blindness to red.   Only the extreme case J is able to match 360° with grey, or rather black.   H saw the 360° red as dark brown, which he afterwards matched with a darkened yellow.   This red, when diluted—which might be called a medium red—he matches with grey.   The others require differing amounts of red, which shows blindness to red, but suggests that the blindness to red is not of so grave a nature as the blindness to green. This would confirm the results obtained from colour naming, that red as a colour was more often recognized than green.   The results of subjects C and D again, however, point to a lesser defect.   Subject I, although he called red black, could not get an equation with the full red disc.   Both discs when rotated appeared grey to him, but the one was more of a drab colour than the other.   Subject F saw both the outer and inner rings red long before he could get them equated.   The equations of A and B are very similar.

(3) *Red = Green*

	Red + White			=	Green + Black		
A							
B							
C							
D							
E							
F							
G	112	+	248	=	140	+	220
H	232	+	128	=	288	+	72 (2 greys)
I	222	+	138	=	66	+	124+170 white
J	360			=	196	+	164

This Table gives striking results. Subjects A to F could not get an equation—surely this means that red and green are visible to them in some measure.[1] Only the four last cases were able to obtain a match. In their final equations the red discs to the normal eye appeared a vivid red and the green discs a vivid green. I had to get white into the green to lighten it and black in, not to make it darker, but to make it "heavier." Note the result of J, which differs from the others in that the red disc did not require dilution. A further equation was obtained with 360° green. In other words, the colour equation could be obtained from him in any proportion. This was not so with the others. This seems to prove once again that there are varying degrees of colour-blindness—even G and H differ from one another. The variations occur, too, apart from any individual idiosyncrasy—and seem to be variations solely of degree.

[1] At least red and green are influencing their sensations to some extent.

(4) *Red = Yellow + Black*

	Red		Yellow + Black			
A						
B						
C						
D						
E						
F						
G						
H	360	=	25	+	335	(2 browns)
I						
J	360	=	36	+	324	

This confirms the results of equation 3, as regards severity of defect. H sees red as dark brown, and these two equations, of H and J, place them at once in the scoterythrous class as described by Myers in his *Experimental Psychology*, where he gives the equation, 360° red = 18° yellow + 342° black. Helmholtz, in the second edition of his *Physiological Optics*, gives a similar equation.[1] Dark red, therefore, appears as a very much darkened yellow, in the cases of these two subjects, almost a black. Subject F almost obtained an equation. The outer ring (the red ring) was red ; the inner ring was red and brown. The brownish tinge could not be eliminated. The other subjects failed completely to match the two discs.

(5) *Green + Red = Black + White*

	Green +	Red +	Blue	= Black +	White
Normal	194 +	113 +	53	= 255 +	105
A	198 +	108·5 +	53·5	= 276·5 +	83·5
B	302·5 +	28 +	29·5	= 240·5 +	119·5
C	198 +	110 +	52	= 269 +	91
D	204·5 +	118·5 +	37	= 264 +	96
E	230 +	130		= 237 +	123
F	155 +	131 +	74	= 275 +	85
G	277 +	83		= 261 +	99
H	192 +	168		= 187 +	173
I	231·5 +	68 +	60·5	= 271 +	89
J	162 +	198		= 279 +	81

N.B.—J can employ any proportion of red and green and get an equation, for he sees both as grey.

[1] 360° sealing wax red = 35° yellow + 325° black.

A green and red disc alone cannot be equated to grey by the normal eye, for there appears, on adjusting, either too much red or too much green. If the green and the red are eliminated, the result is yellow. A third colour, therefore, is necessary before a satisfactory equation can be obtained. This experiment was carried out on 22 normal subjects, and the average of their results gives a fair indication of the normal equation. The equations obtained from the colour-blind subjects show marked deviations in some cases. Six of them required the addition of the blue before they evinced satisfaction, although in 4 cases their final equations appeared defective to the normal eye ; the other 4 were able to obtain a match from the mixture of the red and the green alone.

C and D, as before, gave excellent results. C's match was almost identical with the normal equation.

B, F and I show deviations from the normal. All three declared their match to be perfect. In the cases of B and I the outer ring appeared very green to the experimenter and the inner ring decidedly pink by contrast. Both show an excessive proportion of green,

Normal 194°
B ... 302°
I ... 231°

and a correspondingly small section of red, this seeming to point to the fact that the subjects are more blind to green than to red (this result we have obtained before). B could not get a match with red and green alone, for the outer ring appeared too green and the inner too pink ; yet when blue was added he immediately expressed complete satisfaction, although to the experimenter's eye the green was still in evidence. Subject A also was dissatisfied with red and green alone, but immediately the blue was added an instant change of judgment was given and the discs were claimed to be identical.   Subject F shows an abnormal proportion of blue.

The other four subjects were able to obtain good matches without the addition of a third colour, and all expressed satisfaction with their equations.   Subject J could obtain perfect equations with any proportions of red and green. How is it that this is so, and that other subjects suffering from the same defect are unable to do so ?   The E, G, H show a larger proportion of green than red.

These results thus show considerable divergence and point to different degrees of colour-blindness for red and green respectively.   The first few subjects gave clear evidence of seeing and recognizing red and green.   It might perhaps be added that an anomalous trichromate, who was tested and who could pass Stilling's Tables, gave the following equation :   99° green + 208° red + 53° blue = 280° black + 80° white, which showed her to be red-anomalous.

(6) *Blue + Yellow = Black + White.*

Similar results were obtained with blue and yellow discs, the yellow containing a green tinge.   The normal eye requires to add a third disc of red before a satisfactory match can be obtained.

Blue + Yellow + Red = Black + White

	Blue		Yellow		Red		Black		White
Normal	165	+	147	+	48	=	213	+	147
A	237	+	101	+	22	=	197·5	+	162·5
B	172	+	188		—	=	165	+	195
C	175	+	155	+	30	=	195	+	165
D	192	+	147	+	21	=	236	+	124
E	204	+	156		—	=	240	+	120
F	171	+	189		—	=	238	+	122
G	170	+	190		—	=	240	+	120
H	202	+	158		—	=	236	+	124
I	183	+	177		—	=	219	+	141
J	169	+	191		—	=	199	+	161

Only three subjects required the third disc of blue.
C's and D's equations show great similarity to the normal
as before. A in her equation shows more blue and much
less red than the normal. The other subjects were able
to obtain a satisfactory equation without the addition of
the third disc. Their results show considerable similarity. The green contained in the yellow evidently was not
detected by the examinees and the consequence was a set
of equations which appear entirely faulty when viewed
by the normal eye. B's results are not what might be
expected from the previous results obtained, but he
expressed great satisfaction with the match. He is a
most reliable subject, and always takes great pains with
all his equations, not allowing the smallest difference to
pass unobserved. To subject E the final arrangement
appeared as grey, although the discs appeared respectively
pink and green to the examiner. Subject I called the
two discs blue in the final result represented by his
equation, although, as before, pink and green were clearly
visible.

(7) *Green = Yellow + Black*

The green in this equation was a grass green.

Green = Yellow + Black

A   360 = 278 + 82
B   360 = 223 + 137
C
D
E   cannot get rid of brown tint in yellow.
F   360 = 111 + 249
G   outer circle green, inner red.
H   360 = 240 + 120
I   360 = 186 + 174
J   360 = 194 + 166

These are characteristic equations of colour-blinds. Green is seen as a darkened yellow, and most of the subjects obtained this equation.   C and D as before stand apart.   The green was not tried diluted or perhaps an equation with E and G might have been successful.   Evidently this particular shade of green or perhaps of yellow did not suit their colour scheme.

(8)   *Violet = Blue + Black*

	Violet	=	Blue	+	Black
A	360	=	202	+	158
B					
C					
D					
E	360	=	131	+	229
F	360	=	255	+	105
G	360	=	246	+	114
H	360	=	216	+	144
I	360	=	202	+	158
J	360	=	335	+	25

These again show typical colour-blind equations.   Blue and violet are constantly being confused.   The fact that C and D could not obtain an equation calls for little remark.   C, however, always showed considerable confusion in naming colours when matching them.   Violet and blue were both called shades of blue.   Then when these were rotated simultaneously and after a considerable amount of adjusting had been done, he declared he saw too much green (!) on the outer disc (evidently the red in the violet).   He finally declared the inner disc to be a purer blue, and although still convinced that the two discs represented two shades of blue, he was unable to get them matched.

D likewise called both discs shades of blue, the violet being the darker.   Immediately the discs were rotated on the colour wheel, he called the violet disc no longer blue, but purple.

The fact that B is unable to obtain the equation is a curious one. He confuses blue and violet if presented separately, but when they are rotated he can immediately detect the purple element. The equations show a fair similarity except in the case of J, whose equation is totally different from any of the others in respect of the small proportion of black employed. Does this indicate a blindness to blue or a defect in shade ? The blue disc must have differed in brightness from the violet disc, being considerably lighter if we take the other subjects' equations as valid. The results from the Bradley paper test show that there does exist a deficiency in shade perception. To the subjects who obtained the equation violet appears as a darkened blue ; to J violet appears as a fairly bright blue. On the other hand other tests suggest the other explanation—a weakened sensitivity to blue.

(9) *Orange = Yellow + Black*

Orange = Yellow + Black

A					
B					
C					
D					
E					
F	360	=	117	+	243
G					
H	360	=	92	+	268
I	360	=	89	+	271
J	360	=	90	+	270

The last three equations are very similar ; that of subject F shows more yellow. Orange, therefore, appears as a darkened yellow, much darker than green appears to be, if we compare the results obtained in equation 7. This seems correct, for if the spectrum to the left of the neutral band is seen as shades of yellow, the orange will appear a darker shade of yellow than the green.

Take H's results, for example :

360 red = 25 yellow + 335 black.
360 orange = 92 yellow + 268 black.
360 green = 240 yellow+ 120 black.

The yellow disc employed in all three was the same ; more yellow is required as we pass from red to green.

(10) *Orange=Green*

Orange + White = Green + White

A	45·5	+ 314·5	=	93	+ 267
B	114	+ 246	=	134	+ 226
C	156	+ 204	=	148	+ 212
D					
E	37	+ 323	=	76	+ 284
F					
G					
H	256	+ 104	=	360	
I	257	+ 103	=	360	
J	360	+	=	317	+ 43 black

In the equations of subjects A and E, the orange was so diluted that it appeared as a very, very pale pink, the other disc as a very pale green. The colours in B's discs were more pronounced. C this time obtained an equation, a stronger one as regards colour than B even. In both cases, however, the final discs resembled pale pink and pale green. Subject E could not procure an equation, although he called the outer orange ring green, and the inner ring which was green red. With subject G the outer ring was orange, the inner a grey, and therefore no match could be obtained. It will be noted that the equations of H and I are very similar, although H called his result orange, while I named his green. In both cases the full green disc was matched with a diluted orange. Subject J, as before, has an equation of his own, which totally differs from all others. The full orange disc is matched with a darkened green ; both appeared to him a dark grey.

The equation of magenta and violet was tried, but unsuccessfully. To subject I, for example, the two discs appeared as two shades of blue, the former much darker than the latter, but although both were blues it was impossible to equate them, not because they were of different colours but because the violet appeared a " cheerful " blue, whereas the magenta was of a " washed-out drab " appearance. With subject H an equation of magenta and crimson was tried, but when rotated together they could not be matched, for the blue appeared in the magenta. But when the magenta was matched with a blue or with a violet, it lost its blueness, and became a grey, evidently an example of the operation of Weber's Law.

Colour-mixings are valuable for giving the precise colours which appear similar to a colour-blind, and seem to be a most useful test. The one disadvantage—at least, if used for practical purposes—is the time they require, but for theoretical requirements they are indispensable. Besides giving valuable insight into the individual cases examined, they yield general results in addition.

(1) Each case has been studied by means of the same ten colour mixings ; the same objective tests have been applied, but the subjective results have varied considerably. The outstanding result which appeared with the Holmgren wools and in nomenclature was that the colour defect could be graded. This same result appears decisively here. The subjects at the beginning of the list could not obtain equations which could be procured from those

at the other end.   The extreme cases had no difficulty in matching all the discs, whereas those of the milder type could not possibly accept some of those equations.   Without labouring the point, there is assuredly a clear difference in the degree of defect of all ten subjects.   The less extreme cases *are without doubt influenced by red and green sensations.*

(2) Each case is different from every other case.   While making allowances for grade of defect, there still exists an individuality which marks off each particular case.   A and B, who are very similar in defect, do not always agree in their matches, and the one often fails to equate two colours which have been successfully equated by the other. Subject J seems to have an individuality all his own, which was clearly shown on more than one occasion.

(3) The colour mixings show that in extreme cases, yellow and blue are the two colours from which every other colour is derived.   To quote subject H's results :—

Red	=	25	yellow	+	335 black
Orange	=	92	yellow	+	268 black
Yellow	=				
Green	=	240	yellow	+	120 black
Blue-green	=	167	white	+	193 black
Blue					
Violet	=	216	blue	+	144 black

The above may be taken as the colours of the spectrum. Red, orange, yellow, and green are seen as shades of yellow, the blue-green forms the neutral band ; the rest of the spectrum is seen as shades of blue.

Subject J

Red	=	36	yellow	+	324 black
Orange	=	90	yellow	+	270 black
Yellow					
Green	=	194	yellow	+	166 black
Blue-green	=	111	white	+	249 black
Blue					
Violet	=	335	blue	+	25 black

This result is similar to that of H. In addition, however, this subject matches the same red with 18° white + 342° black. In both cases the red is seen as black. With H the red had to be diluted a little before it was matched with a dark grey.

(4) The following colours are those which may be confused by a red-green colour-blind :

Red with grey, or with black in the case of a shortened spectrum ; blue-green with grey, and red with green ; yellow with orange, and green ; also blue with violet.

(5) The defect seems greater as regards green than as regards red. Otherwise how does one account for 360° green being matched with a grey in the case of A and B for example, whereas the red had to be diluted practically to that required by normal vision before it could be matched with a grey. This agrees with the results from Stilling's Tables, that the red is more often recognized than the green.

(6) Colour-blinds accept as correct equations which can be obtained by the normal eye.

5. Rayleigh's Equation[1]

This is a particular form of colour equation so called after Lord Rayleigh, who by this means was enabled to detect two special forms of variation from the normal, known now as " anomalous trichromates." In matching red and green = yellow, the majority tested centre round a common equation ; there are some, however, who show marked deviation from the normal. The " green anomalous " require a considerably large proportion of green before a match can be obtained, the " red anomalous "

[1] *Nature*, 1881.

require a similarly large proportion of red. The dichromate accepts the normal Rayleigh equation and also marked deviations from the normal.

All subjects were tested with the equation except subject I, from whom, unfortunately, further data could not be obtained.

The results were as follows, and some of them compare quite favourably with the normal :

	Red	+	*Green*	=	*Yellow*	+	*White*	+	*Black*
Normal	197	+	163	=	48	+	48·5	+	263·5
A	184	+	176	=	47	+	52·5	+	260·5
B	181	+	179	=	46	+	48·5	+	265·5
C	186	+	174	=	36	+	65	+	259
D	200	+	160	=	38	+	57	+	265
E	248	+	112	=	27	+	62	+	271
F	187	+	173	=	57	+	47	+	256
G	158	+	202	=	38	+	74	+	248
H	224	+	136	=	32	+	30	+	298
J {	338	+	22	=	35	+			325
{	15	+	345	=	191	+	26	+	143

Anomalous Trichromate

208	+	152	=	44	+	50	+	266

The wide range which is allowed by subject J is remarkable. Unfortunately, the limits in the other matches were not specially noted, but they showed less variation than those of J. D, for example, allowed a variation of about 40 degrees, after which the red was clearly distinguished. A and B and D would permit very little alteration in the proportions. The conclusion we would draw may be aptly expressed in the words of Professor Hayes :—" All the subjects objected to wider extremes of red and green by correctly naming red or green when either one was increased beyond the limits finally decided upon ; they insisted that the mixture was different in quality from the dirty yellow with which it was being matched, no matter how the yellow mixture was varied. Now, since dichromates are supposed to see red and green as yellows, it is difficult to imagine how they were able to detect the reds and greens under the conditions, unless we grant the possibility that they may have some sense of red and green as a colour quality distinct from yellow."[1]

All subjects except H and J recognized the red and green in the two discs, which bears out Professor Hayes' conclusions, and confirms the results previously established.

6. *Analysis of Spectrum*

In the absence of a spectrometer, which was not available for the experiment, we had to resort to testing the subjects with a coloured plate—that in Parsons' *Introduction to Colour-Vision*. A piece of firm paper sufficient to cover the spectrum in its entirety and containing a small vertical aperture was employed. This allowed only a very small part of the spectrum to be seen at one time, and the subject was asked to name the colour visible. This test, without doubt, is open to most serious objections and as a test is not in the least reliable. It is wonderful, therefore, that the results obtained from this primitive spectral exploration agreed with the results obtained from more exact methods.

The following points of the spectrum were taken—they are expressed in Ångström Units.[2]

The wave-lengths are indicated by the presence of Fraunhofer lines which, being constant in position, give a series

---

[1] *American Journal of Psychology*, 1911.
[2] Ångström unit = $\cdot 1\ \mu\mu$.

of fixed points in the spectrum. The colours centre more or less around these points, but the selection of wavelength is to a certain degree arbitrary.

Colours		Å.U.
Black	A —	7606
Dark Red	B —	6869
Red	C —	6564
Orange		
Yellow	D —	5897
Yellow-green		
Green	E —	5271
Blue-green	F —	4862
Blue	G —	4308
Violet	H —	3696
Black		

	Black	Dark Red	Red	Orange	Yellow	Yellow-Green	Green	Blue-Green	Blue	Violet	Black
A	Black	dark red	red	orange	yellow	yellow-green	green	greenish grey	blue	violet	black
B	Black	dark red	red	orange	yellow	yellow-green	green	greenish grey	blue	purple	black
C	Black	brown	red-yellow	orange	yellow	orange	orange	green	blue	dark grey	black
D	very dark blue	dark brown	red	yellow	brown	light yellow	light green	green	blue or green	purple	black
E	Black	reddish grey	red	orange	yellow	light green	grey	greenish grey	light blue	grey	black
F	dark red	dark red	brown	yellowish brown	yellow	brownish yellow	brownish yellow	light red	light red	red	dark red
G	Black	dark red	red	red	yellow	orange	grey	grey	blue	greenish-blue	black
H	Black	dark grey	dark brown	green	yellow	orange	grey	grey	blue	dark grey	black
I	Black	dark red or black	dark red or black	reddish yellow	yellow	reddish yellow or pinkish brown	greenish red	pinkish green	blue	dark blue	blue
J	Black	black	black	medium grey	yellow	grey	medium grey	dark grey	blue	black	black

K

This rough spectral diagnosis is instructive. A glance at J's spectrum reveals the fact that his defect is very grave. He has the spectrum considerably shortened at the red end, for no colour is seen until the sodium or D line is reached ; even the orange is seen as a medium grey. A large neutral band is revealed in the centre, including the yellow-green, the green and the blue-green ; this is larger than is usual, for the yellow-green, too, is merely seen as a brightness. The spectrum at the violet end seems to be shortened, leaving only a narrow band of blue. Joy Jeffries notes that Dr Edward Raehlmann in Halle, when testing for colour-blindness, found that when the red end of the spectrum was shortened the violet end was also reduced—this observation has not been generally confirmed.[1] This subject thus has only two narrow bands of colour in the spectrum—a narrow band of yellow, and one of blue, which would account for the regular unfailing series of greys which all colours appear to him to be. It may further account for the fact that blue is often seen as a grey.

The spectrum of subject I is somewhat different, but from his confused nomenclature it is difficult to determine what spectral colours are visible to him. At the time of being tested his colour-vision had become the centre of interest at home, and he had been instructed in the colours of the spectrum just before he was tested, which was unfortunate for the test. It is evident, however, that he has the red end of the spectrum shortened, but not to such an extent as J. Sensations of colour begin for him about the band of orange. He probably has an extended neutral band, but this would require a more thorough investigation before a definite decision could be reached. Yellow-green he calls reddish yellow or pinkish brown, green he calls greenish red, and blue-green he

---

[1] Raehlmann himself (in *Archiv für Ophthalm.*, Vol. XXII) gives the shortening of both spectral ends as characteristic of the rarest type of colour-blindness.

designates as pinkish green. This shows an entire lack of recognition of the colours. His blue, however, is more extended and reaches well out to the violet end.

Subject H is a third case of a shortened spectrum. His colour sensations begin in the red. He has a large neutral band over the green and blue-green, and he seems to have—as in the case of J—the spectrum shortened at the violet end.

Subject E has not generally been regarded as having a shortened spectrum, for he passed Stilling's Table 3, and in the matches with wools and in nomenclature, he did not give any evidence which might give rise to the belief that a shortened spectrum existed. He was one of the subjects, however, who more than once called a blue a grey, and it would seem here that the violet end of the spectrum is shortened, leaving a narrower band of blue than usual. It will be noticed further that he names the dark red a reddish-grey. He has a neutral band which embraces green and blue-green. Subject C is the only other one who calls the violet, grey; he also calls the dark red a brown, but his nomenclature is so bad that it is an unreliable criterion.

Subject G with a normal length of spectrum has a large neutral band extending over the green and the blue-green. A and B with shortened and unshortened spectrums respectively—if Stilling's Tables are correct—have a grey band in the blue-green. This spectral examination does not show shortened spectrum in the case of A, as one would expect since she was totally unable to read Table 3, of the Pseudoisochromatic Tables of Stilling.

These results amplify the conclusions already reached regarding the difference in degree of the defect. Those cases in which the spectrum is shortened appear to suffer from a greater abnormality of vision than those whose spectrum is of normal length.   The results also raise the question whether when a spectrum is shortened at the red end we may expect in extreme cases a shortening at the violet end as well.   Further, the neutral band varies its position ; sometimes it is in the blue-green, at other times in the green ;   while it occasionally includes both.   In more extreme cases it may extend to the yellow-green.

(7) *Bradley Paper Test*

This test was suggested by Dr Drever.   It was originally devised as a possible means of explaining the term reddish green which, as we have seen, is used by some colour-blinds, but it was found also to give a fairly reliable spectral analysis.   The Bradley colours with shades and tints were arranged in a specific order on two large rectangular oblongs of white cardboard.   The colours in each case measured two inches by one inch.   These were arranged at equal distances apart, nine in a row, five rows in all on each sheet.   The centre rows (called *c* and C respectively) contained the pure spectral and extraspectral colours beginning with violet-red, red, orangered, red-orange, orange, and passing with as many gradations through yellow, green, blue and violet until redviolet was reached.   The two rows above that contained shades 1 and 2 of these colours (shade 1 called *b* and B ; shade 2 called *a* and A).   The two rows below that contained two tints of these colours (tint 1 called *d* and D ; tint 2 called *e* and E).   Looking from left to right, with the two sheets contiguous, there were eighteen vertical columns each containing five colours, comprising tints and shades of a *single* hue.   The total number of colours equalled 90.   A third smaller card contained the ten Bradley shades of black, white and grey.

In addition, 100 oblongs of colour (including shades of grey) were affixed to visiting cards and the position of each relative to the larger card indicated on the back.

The method of procedure might be divided into three parts. (1) The large cardboards containing the colours were spread out in a good light before the examinee. The experimenter picked out at random one of the smaller cards containing a colour or a grey and asked the subjects to match it exactly from the larger assortment before him, with colour and brightness identical. To the normal eye this is simplicity itself, but it was amazing that to the colour-blinds this often proved a task of stupendous difficulty, even although the arrangement of colours in a regular order would seem to offer a little guidance. The arrangement of the colourless series on a separate card did not seem to suggest a difference in sensations either, as the greys, the black and the white were often matched with colours. (2) The subjects were asked to name the colours in the different rows. This gave a good indication of the spectrum as it appeared to them, and considerable insight into their defect. (3) An attempt was made to analyse the colour sensation known as " reddish green."

(1) *The Naming of the Colours*

(2) *Matching Colours*

The second part of the test acted as a confirmatory test to the last one. A larger variety of spectral hues was available, which accordingly gave more accurate results. Although the results are rather lengthy, it will be advisable to record them in full.

On the next page is the Table with the colours as they appear to the normal eye.

	a	b	c	d	e
1	Red-Violet	Violet	Violet-Red	pale Violet	pale Violet
2	very dark Red-Violet	Red-Violet	Red	Red	Pink
3	Red-Violet	dull Red-Orange	Red	pale Pink	pale Pink
4	Bright Red	dull Brown-Red	Red	pale Pink	pale Pink
5	Bright Red	Orange	Orange	pale Orange	pale Pink
6	Red-Orange	light Orange	Orange	pale Yellow-Pink	Yellow-Pink
7	dull Yellow	light Brown-Orange	Yellow	pale Brown-Yellow	pale Brown
8	dull Green	Yellow-Green	pale Yellow	Yellow	Cream
9	Green	Green	Yellow-Green	Yellow-Green	very pale Green

	A	B	C	D	E
1	Green	Yellow-Green	Yellow-Green	pale Yellow-Green	Cream
2	Green	grass Green	Green	pale Green	pale Green
3	Blue-Green	Blue-Green	Blue-Green	pale Blue-Green	pale Blue-Green
4	Blue	Blue	Blue	pale Blue	pale Blue-Green
5	Blue	Blue	Blue	Blue	pale Blue
6	Violet	Violet	royal Blue	pale Violet-Blue	pale Violet
7	Violet	Purple	Purple	pale Violet-Blue	pale Violet
8	dark Purple	dark Purple	Violet	pale Violet	pale Violet
9	very dark Violet	very dark Violet	Red-Violet	pale Blue-Pink	pale Violet

1	Black
2	White
3–10	Shades of Grey

On page 119 are the results of the different subjects. The first two parts of the experiment will be discussed together.

Subject A

	a	b	c	d	e
1	dark Violet	Violet	Violet	Violet	pale Violet
2	dark Red	dark Red	dark Red	Red	Red
3	Red	Red	Red	Red	Pink
4	Red	Red	Red	Red	Pink
5	Red	Red	Orange	Red	Pink
6	Brown	Orange	Orange	Reddish-Yellow	Pink with Yellow
7	Green	Greenish-Yellow	Yellow	Yellow	Yellow
8	Green	Greenish-Yellow	Yellow	Yellow	Yellow
9	Green	Green	Yellow-Green	Yellow	Yellow

	A	B	C	D	E
1	Green	Green	Green	Yellow	Yellow
2	Green	Green	Green	Green	pale Green
3	Green	Green	Green	Green	Blue
4	Blue	Blue	Blue	Blue	Blue
5	Blue	Blue	Blue	Blue	Blue
6	Blue	Purplish	Blue	Blue	Blue
7	Blue	Purplish	Blue	Blue	Blue
8	Blue	Purplish	Violet	Blue	Blue
9	dark Grey	Violet	Violet	Violet	Blue

1	Black	6	Shades of Greenish Grey
2	White	7	do.
3	Grey	8	do.
4	Green	9	do.
5	Greenish Grey	10	do.

The most striking fact about this Table is that the shades of grey are taken to be shades of greenish grey, a clear confusion of green with grey. This confirms all the other experiments that the blindness is more one of green than of red, the only exception, curiously enough, being the Rayleigh equation, where less green than red was employed to match the yellow. A neutral band in the spectrum does not make its appearance in the naming, but later the grey cards are invariably matched with the blue-green, thus indicating a weakened sensitivity in this region. The green in yellow-green is not always recognized but is the colour frequently called yellow. There is also a confusion of blues and violets and purples. One of the red-violets is called a dark grey. This colour is an extra-spectral colour and is the complementary of the blue-green which forms the neutral band. This forms a second neutral band beyond the spectrum. There seems to be no sign of a shortened spectrum.

In matching colours, A made many mistakes particularly with the blue-greens. The most interesting results were obtained by asking the subject to match the grey cards. These she invariably matched with the blue-greens. The white card, too, was thought to be green, and was matched with C3, D3 and E3, blue-green and its two tints. A darker shade of grey she matched with B3 (a shade of blue-green) and when asked to match B3, she looked carefully over all the greys. The darkest shade of grey was matched with the darkest shade of blue-green. This proves conclusively the presence of a blue-green neutral band.

Other matches show a confusion of blues with violets. D8 (a violet) was matched with C4 (a blue).

The perception of shade seems to be good, although mistakes occur here and there. For example, $d2$ is matched with $d2$, $d4$, $b3$ and $b4$; these are all thought to be identical in colour and shade.

Subject B

	a	b	c	d	e
1	Greenish Crimson	Greenish Purple	Purple	Blue-Pink	Pink
2	very dark Crimson	Crimson	Crimson	Red	Red
3	Brown	dark Red	Red	pale Red	Pink
4	light Brown	dark Red	Red	pale Red	Pink
5	light Brown	Red	Orange	pale Red	Yellowish Pink
6	Green	Greenish Red	Orange	Yellow	Yellowish Pink
7	Green	Greenish Red	Yellow	Yellow	Yellow
8	Green	Greenish Red	Yellow	Yellow	Yellow
9	Green	Green	Greenish Yellow	Greenish Yellow	Yellow

	A	B	C	D	E
1	dark Green	Green	grass Green	Greenish Yellow	Yellow
2	dark Green	Green	Green	Green	Greenish White
3	very dark Green	Grey	Blue-Green	Blue-Green	Greenish Blue
4	Blue	Purple	Blue	Blue	Blue
5	Blue	Blue	Blue	Blue	pale Blue
6	Blue	dark Blue	Blue	Blue	pale Blue
7	Blue	Purple	Violet ?	Blue	pale Blue
8	light Blue	Purple	Purple	Blue	Blue with Red
9	Blue Green and Red	dark Purple	Purple	Reddish Blue	Blue with Red

1	Black
2	White
3–10	Different shades of Green

Here again the shades of grey are seen as different shades of green, and there is a suggestion of a neutral band in the blue-green.   The extra-spectral colours give interesting results.   They are evidently puzzling colours. We find they are described as greenish crimson, dark greenish purple, and blue green and red.   The green in the greenish crimson (a dark shade of violet-red) is said to be similar to that of the same shade of the blue-green, which seems a striking coincidence.

This subject seems to have a greater confusion of colours than subject A ; he does not always clearly distinguish between yellows and greens, nor can he always discriminate the reds.

In matching colours, he shows a better perception of shade than A.   His confusion is similar to hers in that greys and blue-greens are constantly mixed.   He also matches one of the extra-spectral colours with C3, the blue-green.

Subject C

	a	b	c	d	e
1	Green or Grey	Green or Grey	Green or Grey	Green or Grey	Green or Grey
2	Brown	Brown	Brown	Brown	Reddish Green
3	Brown	Brown	Brown	Greenish Red	Reddish Green
4	Brown	Brown	Crimson	Greenish Red	Reddish Green
5	Brown	Brown	light Brown	Yellow and light Brown	Yellow and Green
6	Brown	light Brown	light Brown	light Brown	Yellow and Green
7	light Brown	light Brown	Yellow	light Brown	Yellow and Green
8	light Brown	light Brown	Yellow	Yellow	Yellow and Green
9	light Brown	Greenish Brown	Greenish Yellow	light Brown	Yellow and White

	A	B	C	D	E
1	Greenish Brown	Greenish Brown	Greenish Brown	light Brown	Yellow and White
2	Green	Greenish Brown	dark Green	Greenish Brown	Green and White
3	dark Green	Green	light Greenish Grey	Green or Grey	light Green
4	Blue	Blue	Blue	Blue	light Green
5	Blue	Blue	Blue	Blue	light Blue
6	Blue	Blue	Blue	Blue	Blue
7	Blue	Blue	Blue	Blue	Blue
8	Blue	Blue	Blue	Blue	Blue
9	dark Green or Grey	Green	Blue	Blue	Blue

1	Black
2	White
3–10	Grey or Green

This Table emphasizes the serious features of C's defect. We have already seen how his nomenclature is at variance with his colour equations. This is a further proof of the curiously contradictory results which the diagnosis of his case reveals.

There evidently exists a blue-green neutral band, with the complementary purple also seen as grey. All the hues of violet-red and some of those of red-violet he calls grey or green, and compares them with the grey cards as being of a similar nature. He has a well-marked confusion of blue and violet ; he only mentions red once (crimson), except when he uses the term in the compound phrase, reddish green. This would seem to indicate either a deficiency in red, or an extremely bad nomenclature. The term orange, too, is never mentioned ; brown takes the place of it and red.

In colour matching he shows great confusion in shade

as well as in colour. A dark grey which he thought was a green was matched with $d1$, a pale violet ; $e1$, a similar colour, was matched with a grey. These two colours belong to the extra-spectral neutral band of grey. A8, a dark purple, was matched with B1, a yellow-green, and also with $a6$, $a8$, $a9$, orange and greens. B8, of the same hue, was matched with a lighter shade of yellow-green. For $d5$, an orange colour, no match could be found, and the subject could not even remember the name of the colour. He later described it when going over the colours as composed of yellow and light brown. He was rarely content with giving one match to a colour, but frequently gave three or four, showing a defect in shade,

e.g., A8 = $a6$, $a8$, $a9$, B1.
B8 = B4, B8, $b8$, C8.
$b7$ = $b7$, $b8$, $c5$, $c6$.

It is difficult to reconcile these results with the results obtained from him in his colour equations, but they do correspond with the other tests we have considered.

Subject D

	a	b	c	d	e
1	not Purple	Purple	Purple	Purple	Purple
2	dark Brown	dark Brown	dark Grey	dark Brown	dark Brown
3	Brown	Brown	light Red	Red	Brown
4	Brown	Brown	Red	Red	Brown
5	Brown	Yellow	Brown	light Yellow	Brown
6	Yellow	Brown	Yellow	Brown	Brown
7	Brown	Brown	Brown	Yellow	Brown
8	Green	Green or Yellow	Yellow	Yellow	Yellow
9	Green	Green	Green	Brown Yellow or Green	Yellow

	A	B	C	D	E
1	Green	Green	Green	Green	very light Green
2	Green	Green	dark Green	Green	very light Green
3	Green	Green or Blue	pale Blue	very light Green	Blue
4	Blue	Blue	light Blue	Blue	Blue
5	Blue	Blue	Blue	Blue	Blue
6	Purple	Blue	Blue	Purple	Blue
7	Purple	Purple	Purple	Purple	Blue
8	Purple	Purple	dark Purple	Purple	Purple
9	Brown	Purple	Purple	Purple	Purple

1	Black
2	White
3–10	Shades of Grey

This Table calls for little comment. It seems to suggest a neutral band of red, for red is seen as a dark grey. Further, orange is not recognized throughout. A confusion of red with brown and of yellow with green is also shown. It also reveals difficulty with the purples, and some doubt in naming them. In the pale tints in row e, he sees no pink at all, but names them brown; $d9$, a yellow, is described as a brown, or yellow, or green. He would appear to be better classed as an anomalous trichromate, and not as a colour-blind, had not the acceptance of the Rayleigh equation proved otherwise. He is certainly a " dangerous " colour-blind so far as practical occupations go.

In matching colours he shows a slight defect in shade, and at times is unable to obtain a match to satisfy him. For example, in matching $c9$, he states that $c9$ is too dark and $d9$ too light—the exact match lies between these two. $a6$ is matched with $a5$, $a4$, $b4$, $b3$.

One match which tends to suggest a neutral band in

the extra-spectral purple is the match used with c_1. c_1 is technically known as a violet red, but it was matched with c_9, a yellow-green. This is the same colour which he could not describe, and about which he could only state that it was not a purple. This may indicate the existence of a small band of the spectrum in which green is not visible, and further it may suggest that the yellow spreads out into the yellow-green, for it is always about that region that mistakes occur. It is an interesting case which would repay further study by more exact methods.

Subject E

	a	b	c	d	e
1	very dark Grey almost Black	dark Blue almost Black	Blue and Red	Pink	Pink
2	very dark Red almost Black	dark Red	dark Red	Red	light Red
3	dark Red	Red	Red	light Red	Flesh
4	dark Red	Red	Red	light Red	light Red
5	Bright Red	Brighter Red	Orange	Red	Red
6	Brown	light Brown	Orange	Red and Yellow	Red and Yellow
7	Bright Green	light Brown	Yellow	Bright Yellow	light Yellow
8	Green	light Brown	Yellow	Yellow	Yellow
9	Green	Green	Bright Green	Green	Yellow and Green

	A	B	C	D	E
1	Green	Green	Green	Green	almost White
2	Grey	Grey Green	dark Green	Green	Grey Green
3	dark Grey	Grey	Grey	Grey	light Grey
4	Blue	Blue	Blue	Blue	Blue
5	Blue	Blue	Blue	Blue	Blue
6	Blue	Blue	Blue	Blue	Blue
7	Blue	Blue	Blue	Blue	Blue
8	Blue	Blue	Blue	Blue	Blue
9	Blue	Black	Blue	Blue	Blue

1	Black		3–9	Shades of Grey
2	White		10	Grey Green

This Table clearly reveals a neutral band in the green and the blue-green, which confirms the diagnosis of the previous test. The two shades of red-violet and violet-red appear as almost black, revealing a second neutral band there. The violets themselves are not recognized, but all are considered as shades of blue. Red, orange and yellow are discriminated as colours, although occasionally they overlap and the change of colour, as seen by the normal eye, is delayed in his case. It is only in the centre row that he recognizes orange—to the tints and shades the term is not applied, although he twice uses the expression red and yellow; $a7$, seen by the normal eye as a dull yellow, the subject describes as a bright green. While the greys appear as such, the darkest shade is thought to be a green.

In matching colours, considerable confusion is revealed with the greys. Shades 3, 5, 7 and 8 are all matched with C3, the blue-green. This occurred with most of the subjects. Shade 6 is matched with B3, a blue-green. Shade 9 is matched with $c2$, $a3$, $b3$, $a5$; that is, with red and shades of red. This shows a confusion of red and grey—a conclusion we have previously reached. Shade 10, which is to him a dark green, is matched with A3 and B3, two shades of blue-green.

A3, a blue-green, which he considers to be a grey containing red, is matched correctly, but only after all the reds have been carefully examined. A4, a blue to the normal eye (though technically a tint of green-blue) is matched with $a4$, $a5$, $b3$, $b4$, shades of red and orange. A9, a very dark violet, is matched with A9, B9, $b1$, and A1; $b1$ is the other extra-spectral colour and A1 a green, which all appear as grey. This explains why purples, greens and greys are considered as correct matches. It may also

explain why some violets or purples were seen as grey in
some of the previous experiments.

Subject F

	a	b	c	d	e
1	Red	Red	Reddish Blue	Reddish Blue	light Red
2	Red	Red	Red	Red	Red
3	Red	Red	Red	Reddish Green	Green
4	Red	Red	Red	Green	Green
5	Red	Reddish Brown	Reddish Brown	Yellowish Brown	? Green in it
6	Reddish Brown	Reddish Brown	Yellow	Yellow	Yellow
7	Yellowish Brown	Yellow	Yellow	Yellow	Yellow
8	Yellowish Brown	Yellow	Yellow	Yellow	Yellow
9	Yellowish Brown	Yellow	Yellow	Yellow	Yellow

	A	B	C	D	E
1	Reddish Brown	Reddish Brown	Yellow	Yellow	Yellow
2	Reddish Brown	Reddish Brown	Yellowish Brown	Yellowish Green	Grey
3	Red	Red	Greenish Grey	Reddish Green	light Green ?
4	Reddish Blue	Reddish Blue	Blue	Blue	Reddish Blue
5	Blue	Blue	Blue	Blue	Blue
6	Blue	Blue	Blue	Blue	Blue
7	Blue	Blue	Blue	Blue	Blue
8	Blue	Blue	Blue	Blue	Blue
9	Blue	Red	Blue	Blue	Blue

1	Black	6	Red
2	White	7	Grey
3	Reddish Green	8	Reddish Green
4	Reddish Green	9	Grey
5	Red	10	Green

Much confusion is exhibited between the red and green in this Table. The green sensation is weakened in the green and the blue-green ; whether there is a complete neutral band here is doubtful—but there is a possibility that such is the case. Certainly, the green is not a clearly defined sensation for him. It is curious, too, how often a green oblong is named red by the subject. Usually with F a green is confused with yellow, but in this instance there is a direct confusion with red. In columns A and B, green is never mentioned, but its place is taken by a yellowish and a reddish brown. $e3$ and $e4$, two pale pinks, are both termed greens ; E3, however, a green, is recognized as such, but some other colour unknown is also present. The darker tint of the same green is described as a reddish green.

Violet is seen as blue throughout. The shades of grey appear as greys, reds, greens and reddish greens. The complete confusion of reds and greens with each other, and with grey, seems to be indicated in this instance.

Matching colours reveals a good perception of shade. The white card was matched with E3, a very pale blue-green, and grey was matched with C3, also a blue-green. $e1$, an extra-spectral purple, was matched with E4, another pale blue-green. This is evidently a characteristic of some colour-blinds. E8, a pale violet, was matched with $e1$ and $d4$, a purple and a pale pink. This is the typical confusion of blue with pink. $a7$, a dull yellow, and C2, a green, were judged to be identical.

It is worthy of note that the violet-reds are described as reddish blues, a relatively correct description, but the fact becomes really significant, when we find that green-blues are similarly described.

L

Subject G

	a	b	c	d	e
1	? dark Crimson	dark Grey	Violet	Grey	Grey or Green
2	Crimson	Crimson	Crimson	Red	Red
3	Red	Red	Red	Red	very pale Red
4	Red	Red	Red	Red	Green
5	Red	Red	Red	Red and Yellow	Green
6	Green	Green	Green	Red and more Yellow	Green
7	Green	Green	Yellow	Yellowish Green	Greenish Yellow
8	Green	Green	Yellow	Yellow	Yellowish Green
9	Green	Green	Green	Green	Yellowish Green

	A	B	C	D	E
1	Green	Green	Green	Green	Cream
2	Green	Green	Green	Grey	Grey
3	Grey	Grey	Grey	Grey	Bluish Grey
4	Blue	Blue	Blue	Blue	Bluish Grey
5	Blue	Blue	Blue	Blue	Blue
6	not so Blue	Blue	Blue	Blue	Blue
7	Blue	Blue	Blue	Blue	Blue
8	Blue	Blue	Red and Blue	Blue	Blue
9	Grey	Grey	Blue	Blue	Blue

1	Black
2	White
3–10	Green

As in previous cases, the neutral band in the blue-green is strongly marked, but it extends into the green as well. The purples present great difficulty, and are sometimes called grey, sometimes green. Orange is not recognized, but is replaced by green; e4 and e5, pale pinks, are described as greens. To the right of the neutral band the spectrum is seen as shades of blue. The shades of grey are not discriminated from shades of green.

In matching, the white card is confused with E3, a very pale blue-green, the greys likewise. c9, a yellow-green, is not differentiated from C4, a green-blue. There is, too, frequent confusion between yellows and yellow-greens.

Subject H

	a	b	c	d	e
1	Black	Blue	dark Blue	Blue	light Blue
2	dark Brown (Black)	Brown	dark Brown (Black)	medium Brown	medium Brown
3	dark Brown	Brown	dark Brown	Grey	Grey
4	light Brown	Brown	light Brown	Grey	Grey
5	light Brown	Brown	light Brown	Grey	Grey
6	very light Brown	light Brown	very light Brown	light Grey	dirty Yellow
7	very light Brown	Orange	Orange	Yellow	dirty Yellow
8	very light Brown	dark Orange	light Orange	Yellow	light Yellow
9	very light Brown	dark Orange	dark Orange	dark Yellow	light Yellow

	A	B	C	D	E
1	Brown	light Brown	Orange	light Yellow	White
2	medium Brown	light Brown	medium Brown	Grey	dirty White
3	Grey	very dark Grey	dark Grey	Grey	light Grey
4	dark Blue-Grey	dark Blue	dark Blue	Blue	dark Grey
5	dark Blue	vivid Blue	dark Blue	Blue	Blue
6	very dark Blue	Blue	very dark Blue	Blue	Blue
7	dark Blue	Blue	very dark Grey	Blue	Blue
8	dark Blue	Blue	very dark Grey	Blue	light Blue
9	Black	Black	Blue	Blue	light Blue

1	Black
2	White
3–10	Shades of Grey

This Table is an interesting one, for it plainly shows the effect of a shortened spectrum. The neutral band embraces the green and the blue-green, and is present in the unsaturated green-blues. This will account for the fact that certain blues in the wool test were considered greys. Very pale tints of this colour or very dark shades will be so confused.

The complementary colour of the blue-greens is seen as blue or black—the shades as black, the tints as blue. The tint which appears as a bluish pink to the normal eye is composed of red and violet. As the subject is blind to red, the red sensation is completely absent, and the violet sensation remains, which is described as blue.

Red is seen as black or very dark brown, and, if we consider row c, this colour name serves to describe all the red and the orange sensations. No colour is recognized until the orange-yellow ($c7$) is reached. This is called orange by the examinee, and the same name includes pure yellow, green-yellow, and yellow-green. "Orange" is constantly applied to a green containing yellow.

The tints show markedly the absence of a red sensation, for $d3$, $d4$, $d5$, and $d6$ yield only greys.

One other interesting feature is worthy of note. C7 and C8, a blue violet and a violet respectively, are colourless, which points to a shortening of the violet end of the spectrum. This coincides with the finding in the last experiment.

In matching, many points of interest came to light. The black card was matched with red ($c2$), the white with a very pale blue-green (E3). Certain shades of grey were confused with $e2$, $e3$ and $c3$, reds and pinks; others were thought to be identical with the blue-greens. The general mistakes made with the colours were blues, erroneously judged to be violets, and yellows, greens.

A defect in shade, though not a serious one, occurs frequently.

e.g., B7 and C8
        D1 ,, *d*9
        A4 ,, B6
        E9 ,, E7
        *b*4 ,, *d*5

In these cases the colour is correct, but the shade is wrong.

Subject J

	a	b	c	d	e
1	Grey	Grey	Blue tinge	Blue tinge	Grey
2	Black	Black	Black	Black	Grey
3	Grey	Grey	Grey	Grey	Grey
4	Grey	Grey	Grey	Grey	Grey
5	Grey	Grey	Grey	Grey	Grey
6	Grey	Grey	Orange	Grey	Grey
7	Grey	Grey	Yellow	Orange	Yellow
8	Grey	Grey	Yellow	Yellow	Yellow
9	Grey	Grey	Yellow	Yellow	light Yellow

	A	B	C	D	E
1	Grey	Grey	Grey	Yellow	White
2	Grey	Grey	Grey	Grey	Grey
3	Grey	Grey	Grey	Grey	faint Blue
4	Blue	Blue	Blue	Blue	Blue
5	Blue	Blue	Blue	Blue	Blue
6	Blue	Blue	Blue	Blue	Blue
7	Blue	Blue	Blue	Blue	Blue
8	Blue	Blue	Blue	Blue	Blue
9	Black	Black	Blue	Blue	Blue

1	Black
2	White
3-10	Grey

This was a most difficult test for this subject, and caused him intense fatigue, so that he had to rest his eyes frequently.

This Table presents different features from any of the others, for it reveals an amazing lack of colour sensation. The spectrum is shortened and no colour is seen before the yellow-orange (*c*6). With the last subject, the colours beyond that were named brown, but with this subject they are merely brightnesses. The yellow band in the two shades is non-existent, and only grey is seen until the blue begins to make an impression, which indicates a weakened sensitivity to yellow. The neutral band is large, extending over the yellow-green, the green, and the blue-green. His spectrum accordingly is as follows :— A shortened spectrum at the red end ; a large grey band ; a patch of yellow ; a neutral central band, larger than ordinary ; and then a region of blue which seems here to extend to the violet. The last test pointed to shortening at the violet end.

In matching colours marked confusion was revealed, which was to be expected, considering the large number of colours which the subject sees as grey. This part of the experiment was lengthy because J had to search all the cards each time.

Black was matched with *a*2, *a*3, *b*2, *c*2, *d*2, all reds, which is a typical feature of his case. White was matched with *e*8, E3, E4, a cream colour and two very pale blue-greens. No. 4, a shade of grey, was confused with *b*4, *c*4, *e*2, orange red, red and pink, and with A2 and B3, green and blue-green. No. 7, a different shade of grey, was matched with *a*9, *b*5, B1, C3, *c*4, *d*3, *e*2, all of which were claimed to be identical with the test card. They include green, orange, yellow-green, red, blue-green, pink. No. 9, a dark shade of grey, was not differentiated from *e*2, *b*3, *d*3, *b*4, *c*4, B3, pinks, reddish-orange, red and blue-green.

It will be noticed from these few examples that there exists a decided defect in shade perception, which seems to be caused by the shortening of the spectrum.

In matching colours the same confusion exists, and all are characterized by the large selection made.

d1, a tint of red violet, was found to be a most difficult test, for it did not appear as a pure blue. It was finally matched with d1, c1, C9, as well as with B4, a blue. c6, an orange, was matched with the following large variety, c6, c5, b6, b7, a7, a8, a9, B1, B2, A2, shades of orange, yellow and green. C5, a blue, yielded also an interesting, assortment of colours. It was matched correctly and with different shades of the same colour, but placed with it were greens and pinks, giving a total of eight in all. This includes the typical confusion of blues and pinks. Very often the extra-spectral colours are matched with blue, and the inevitable confusion of blue with violet constantly occurs.

This experiment confirmed some of the facts previously noted in the other tests.

(1) It has shown clearly the difference in degree of the colour-blindness of the ten subjects, and suggested the reason why. In the case of J, it was seen that the yellow and blue bands of the spectrum were very small in extent compared with the other subjects. His neutral band in the centre was broader, comprising yellow-green, green and blue-green. H's neutral band extended over the green and blue-green only, likewise subject E. In the milder cases, the blue-green was the sole region affected. The extent of the neutral band must, therefore, be a factor determining the degree of defect. If the blue-green alone is affected, then the green appears to be seen either as yellow or as green.

(2) A neutral band at the red end of the spectrum, as H and J have, seems to be associated with a defect of a graver character.

(3) The most abnormal cases recorded are those with shortened spectrum, except in the case of A, who, according to Stilling's Tables, has a shortened spectrum, but who

shows little evidence of it apart from confusing blues and pinks.

(4) It appears that a shortened spectrum is associated with a defect in perception of shade. This is evident with H and J.

(5) A second neutral band occurs beyond the spectrum in the purples.

(6) Although a colour may be recognized by a colour-blind, it may, when mixed with white or black, undergo a change in hue imperceptible to the normal eye, but which will cause it to be placed in a different category by the colour-blind.

3.   The Colour Sensation of Reddish Green

Reddish green is a term much employed by colour-blinds, but it does not seem to be characteristic of all cases. H and J do not use the term at all. This may mean that it is not common in severe cases of colour-blindness, but is only employed where the defect is milder. Edridge-Green explains it from the point of view that the term belongs to the three-unit class, those who can see red, green and violet. Reddish green is the term applied to the colour seen at the junction of their red and their green. It is not a pure red nor is it a pure green, and the best description of it seems to be in terms of both colours. This is quite a sound explanation, and meets the facts, if the theory of Edridge-Green is accepted. If we, for a moment, place subject B among the three-unit class, and admit that he can distinguish three colours in the spectrum, then the explanation seems quite feasible. But one characteristic of the three-unit class is that red and green are never confused.[1] This does not apply to B, for he often mistakes the one colour

---

[1] Unless under very special circumstances.

for the other. The fact necessarily excludes him from the three-unit class, and the explanation no longer applies.

Peddie, in his recent book on *Colour-Vision*, seems to attribute this term to special cases of trichromatic vision. He is an adherent of the Young-Helmholtz theory, and accepts the three fundamental colours, red, green and blue as forming the three apices of the colour triangle. There may exist a case in which the red and the blue remain unaltered, while the green becomes the yellow complementary to the blue. In other words, the lower half of the absolute triangle becomes 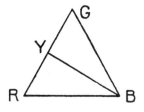 the colour triangle. Two of the fundamental colours are still " simple " colours, the third has become a " fused " colour—yellow, which is nevertheless by training called green, and is stimulated by the wave-lengths which normally stimulate green. So the identical stimulations, which normally extend over the spectrum range red to yellow, now extend from red to green ; and the double colour characteristics of the intermediate yellow-reds or red-yellows now extend from red to green. The compulsory change in nomenclature is, therefore, found by replacing " yellow " by " green." Thus arise the " red-greens " of some trichromatic eyes.[1]

Let us now consider what colours have been called reddish-green by the colour-blind.

It is noteworthy that the term was never employed by certain of the subjects, and these subjects are not confined to one extreme. They are A, D, G, H, and J. The two extreme cases, A and J, do not use this term to describe

[1] pp. 67–8.

any colour. B, C, E, F, and I have all, at one time or another, made use of this phrase.

Subject B

In Stilling's Tables he twice used this phrase, once to describe a mole colour, which he called a reddish green, and once to describe a pink, which he called a greenish red. In the Bradley papers test, he used this expression, too. $b6$, $b7$, and $b8$, which are shades 1 of yellow-orange, orange-yellow, and yellow respectively, and which appear to the normal eye as cinnamon brown, brownish orange, and yellowish olive-green, were called greenish reds. In row c, however, there were no greenish reds, but the corresponding colours were termed orange, yellow and yellow. The name was reserved, therefore, for the shades. The orange-yellow, etc., could be explained along Peddie's line.

$a1$, $b1$, and A9, the extra-spectral purples, are called greenish crimson, dark greenish purple, and blue green and red, respectively. The green in $a1$ is said to be similar to the green in A3, which is tint 2 of the blue-green which forms the neutral band of this subject. There seems, one might tentatively suggest, a connection of the neutral band with this phrase. Part of the colour circle outside the spectrum forms a neutral band, as we have seen, complementary to the blue-green. It seems to be that the grey of the neutral band is being called green, and the violet element mixed with the red appears as an impure blue which cannot be called a pure blue, for it does not correspond with the subject's customary sensation of that colour, and in consequence is termed a red, producing the compound colour, red-green. This may occur, therefore, at the junction of the neutral band and the adjoining colours. These same colours were thought to be grey or green by a number of those examined. If B can distinguish some colour element which J, for example, cannot distinguish, and if he designates as green the part which J sees, then he uses the double term to express this compound sensation which he is experiencing. He described A9, as composed of blue, red and green, but B9, a lighter shade of A9, appeared a dark purple, and he refused to admit the presence of a green in it. To the subject, therefore, A9 contained something which B9 did not contain, although to the normal eye there is no indication of any colour change. There must be some definite sensation which is giving rise to the addition of green by the subject.

With the Edridge-Green Lantern B saw the pure green glass as a reddish green. On being asked to match the glass with a skein of wool, he chose a pinkish yellow. This skein appeared green to him, but contained some other colour as well, probably a red, and so the colour as a whole was described as reddish green.

With this subject two different colours have been described as greenish red.

(1) The region between the yellow-orange and the yellow.

(2) The purples.

Subject C

This subject called a number of the Holmgren wools reddish green, or at least red and green.

rose pink	green with red about it
pink	green and red
pale crimson	reddish green
bluish pink	red and green
bluish pink	red and green
bluish red	red and green
pale green	green and red
pale green-blue	red and green

In the case of the bluish pinks it may be incidental to his nomenclature. The blue is named red, the pink, green, and the combined result is a red-green. But that does not explain the pinks nor the greens. With the Bradley papers he placed the reddish greens in the region of the orange, which would seem to agree with Peddie's and Edridge-Green's results. $d3$ and $d4$, tints of orange-red and red-orange, were both termed greenish reds, and $e4$ was described as a lighter shade of greenish red. $e2$, a pink, was also designated a reddish green.

Subject B and C do not always use the phrase to describe the same objective colour stimulus. B employs the term seemingly for dark colours (shades), and C for light colours (tints).

Subject I

Subject I was not tested with the Bradley papers, but with Holmgren's wools; he described a very dark purple as pinkish-greenish-brownish, and a grey likewise. This again seems to connect the neutral band with the term. In the spectrum he called green greenish red, and blue-green pinkish green, which once more is a description of the neutral band in terms of the compound phrase.

Subject E

He only once used this phrase to describe a pale blue as " green with pink in it."

Subject F

In the Bradley papers, $d3$ a tint of orange, was said to be a reddish green; D3, a tint of blue-green, likewise. Some of the greys, which later were matched with the blue-greens, were described as reddish greens.

From the results given by these different subjects

there seem to be three specific kinds of colour experience which are called reddish-greens ; the neutral band of the spectrum, the neutral band beyond the spectrum, and somewhere in the vicinity of the orange region. The phrase is not used by all the subjects, but only by those whom we have constantly maintained are not limiting cases of dichromasy. If our suggestion is correct, that colour-blinds can see red and green in certain circumstances, then the orange is explained along the two cited lines of explanation, namely, that of Peddie and Edridge-Green. The subjects are not to be classed, however, as abnormal trichromates nor as belonging to the three-unit class. They do not see red as normals do, nor green as normals do, but are blind to both colours ; on certain occasions they may recognize one or the other, and the intermediate sensation becomes a reddish green.

8. *Contrast Experiments*

Since Stilling suggested that contrast colours might be used as a suitable test of colour-blindness, various devices have been adopted. Three contrast tests were utilized here.

(*a*) Coloured Shadows

To produce coloured shadows, a lantern was focussed on a white screen. Coloured glasses of red, green, blue and yellow respectively, were introduced in turn, and the coloured light thrown on to the screen. A second source of light was provided by an electric lamp suitably placed. If a pencil is interposed between the lantern and the coloured screen, the rays are cut off and the area of the pencil is illuminated solely by the white light from the lamp, and assumes the complementary colour of its surroundings. The colour-blind is asked to identify the colour of the shadow of the interposed pencil. (The natural light from both sources contained a great number of yellow rays.)

(*b*) Rings Contrast

Stiff paper discs are employed, each disc is divided into three parts, an inner area of colour and an outer area of the same colour. Interposed between them is a narrower ring of black and white which, when rotated, yields a sensation of grey. The grey ring assumes, on the colour mixer, the complementary colour of its surrounding areas.

(*c*) Negative After-Images

The colours red, green, yellow, blue, orange, violet, were cut " W " shape out of Bradley paper. A small pencil mark in the centre of the stimulus colour served as a point of fixation, and was placed over a corresponding pencil mark made on the paper beneath. The time of stimulation varied slightly with different subjects. At a given signal the subject fixated the mark and, after 20 to 30 seconds had elapsed, the stimulus was removed by the experimenter and the after-image appeared on the white paper beneath.

(*a*) Coloured Shadows

The coloured glasses used were blue, yellow, red, and green. They were presented in irregular order in a series of twelve. The results are shown collected together for each subject. The colour of the shadow appears within the bracket, and it was this colour the subject was asked to name.

	Red (Green)	Green (Red)	Blue (Yellow)	Yellow (Blue)
A	Red	Red	Green	Pinkish-Red
B	Blue-Green	Purple	Greenish-Yellowish-Brown	Blue
C	Grey	Grey	light Brown	Blue
D	Green	Yellow	Yellow	Blue
E	Green	Red	light Brown	Blue
F	Red	Red	Yellowish-Brown	dark Red
G	Blue	Blue	Green	Blue
H	Grey	dark Grey or Black	Orange	dark Blue
J	Grey	Grey	Grey	Blue

The subjects have responded to the test in different ways. The green shadow was only recognized as such by B, D, and E. A failed to recognize the green, and confused it with red ; C, H, and J failed to discern any colour, a grey shadow being all that was visible to them. G called it blue—this may be because the red is seen as a grey, but the blue rays in the shadow—caused by the yellow rays from the source of light—remain. This also explains the blue-green of B.

The response to the red shadow shows slightly different results. A and B both recognize the colour, and B discriminates as before the blue element, which makes him describe the sensation as purple. A always seems to recognize red better than she does green. The red is identified, too, by E and F. D calls it yellow and G blue. The latter cannot be explained as a confusion of red and blue, for that is not characteristic of G's case. It is more probable that the same explanation holds as in the response to green, that the red element is not visible in the shadow, and only the strong blue rays remain. The double shadows, which can be seen simultaneously if the pencil approaches the screen, and which appear red and green respectively, are both seen as blue by this subject. C, H, and J see nothing but grey. This test reveals C's weakness, for he does much worse in it than he did in the wool test. To H the red appears almost black ; his shortened spectrum accounts for this.

Yellow is clearly visible to most subjects, although A, B and G call it green. This, as we have previously shown, is a very common confusion. The shadow is seen as brown by E, and yellowish-brown by F, which is a favourite colour name of the latter. H describes it in terms of *his* favourite name, orange. J is the only one of the subjects who fails to experience a colour sensation ; and this fact —that the yellow appears grey—indicates once more a weakened sensitivity.

The blue shadow is more clearly seen by all, although two subjects mistake it for red.

This experiment showed the characteristic defects of the examinees and proved quite satisfactory. It points to a better discrimination of red than green in the case of some of the subjects. J, as before, must be regarded as an extreme case, with H a close second coming next— although H has a decidedly better colour system than J. The other subjects, excepting C and G, in this case, are affected by the stimulation of red and green lights, and their results seem to show some cognizance of these two colours.

(*b*) Rings Contrast

The contrast colour is bracketed as before. It was this colour the subjects were asked to name.

	Red (Green)	Green (Pink)	Blue (Yellow)
A	Grey	Red	Brownish
B	Bluish-Green	Purple	Green
C	Grey	Grey	Green
D	Grey	Grey	Grey
E	Greenish-Grey	Grey	Brownish-Grey
F	Red	Red	Reddish-Brown
G	Grey	Grey	Grey
H	dark Grey	Blue	dark Grey
J	light Grey	light Blue	medium Grey

The stimuli as in the shadow experiment gave varied results. A once more failed to perceive the green, although the red was clearly visible. B, as before, termed the green and red, bluish-green and purple respectively. He is the only subject who can distinguish the two colours. C sees both red and green as grey ; D, usually able to distinguish colours, is not successful this time, for both appear colourless to him. With E, the green only is recognized ; with F, the red only. G, H, and J fail to see both colours. It is curious that H and J both thought the red colour to be blue.

The yellow was not too distinct a colour, and resembled a brown more than a yellow. Some subjects have called it brown, some green, one red, and four grey, including the last three subjects.

(c) After-Images

The colour of the stimuli is given along the top of the columns—the after-image in brackets. (See page 146.)

The blue and yellow after-images are clearly seen by all the subjects, if we overlook the fact that F calls the blue image blue or red. The after-images of the orange and the violet appear distinctly also, even to subject J. It is

M

	Yellow (Blue)	Blue (Yellow)	Red (Green)	Green (Red)	Orange (Blue-Green)	Violet (Yellow)
A	Blue	Yellow	White	Pink	pale Blue	Yellow
B	Blue	Yellow	almost White very pale Green	? Pink very pale	Blue-Green	Yellow
C	Blue	Yellow	Grey	Grey	Blue	Yellow
D	Blue	Yellow	Green	Red	Blue	Yellow
E	light Blue	Yellow	Grey	Grey	light Blue	Yellow
F	Blue or Red	Yellow	White	Blue	Blue	light Brown
G	pale Blue	Yellow	White	White	pale Blue	Yellow
H	Blue	Yellow	Grey	Grey	Blue	Yellow
J	light Blue	Yellow	light Grey almost White	medium Grey	very light Blue	Yellow

instructive to note that B is the only one who calls the after-image blue-green.

When we consider the red and green after-images, a different result makes its appearance. Subject B alone sees the colours correctly, and he is very doubtful what his sensations are, for they are very pale, approaching white. In the case of subject A the red stimulus cannot give her an after-image of green, but the green makes sufficient impression to give her an after-image of red. This confirms the previous conclusions that the blindness to green is greater than that to red.[1] C, E, F, G, H, and J fail to perceive any sensation.

This test is instructive when supplementary. Alone it is unreliable, for there is no objective control.

---

[1] *Cf.* F. Schumann's report of his own case at the First Congress for Experimental Psychology, held at Giessen, 1904. Also article by Ferree and Rand, *Journal of Experimental Psychology*, Vol. II, No. 4, 1917.

CHAPTER V

TESTS AND RESULTS (*concluded*)

9. *The Nagel Card Test*[1]

There are two sets of cards ; 16 marked A, 4 marked B. The procedure differs slightly in the two cases.

In section A the 16 cards are spread out in good day-light illumination. The subject stands upright before the table, on which lie the cards ; he is not allowed to pick them up nor examine the cards at close range, but is asked to indicate his answers by pointing to the cards he selects. Each card contains a circle of variously-coloured dots.

Four questions are asked :

(1) On which cards are there red or reddish spots ? (This does not exclude other colours being present also.)

(2) On which cards are there red spots only ?

(3) On which cards are there green spots only ?

(4) On which cards are there grey spots only ?

In question 1, for example, most colour-blinds select cards 6 or 11 or 12, as containing red spots ; they mistake the yellowish-green and the brown which these contain for red. These errors, Nagel states, are almost complete evidence of colour-blindness. The anomalous trichro-mates, on the other hand, are usually able to pass this test successfully as well as number 2, but they come to grief in questions 3 and 4.

In section B, the colour-blind is asked to designate each colour he sees on the cards. This is not intended as a test of fine discrimination, but is merely to ascertain if

---

[1] 7th Edition.

red can be distinguished from green, or if these are confused with some other colour. A mistake in B1 only is no criterion of colour-blindness, although it may indicate colour anomaly of some kind ; the other cards must also show deficiency before we diagnose colour-blindness.

1.   Red or Reddish Spots

Correct	1	2	3	4		6	7	8	9	10	11	12	13	14	15	16
A		2	3	4			7	8				12			15	16
B	1	2	3					8			11				15	16
C											11					
D	1														15	16
E	1	2	3				7	8		10	11	12		14	15	16
F	1	2	3	4		6	7		9	10	11	12	13	14	15	16
G							7								15	
H	None															
J						6						12				

Section A was found to be a most satisfactory test for all the subjects.

The results divide the subjects into two groups : (1) those who are able to select a number of cards, and (2) those who find few or no cards containing the colours they are looking for. These two groups divide the subjects almost equally according to the order in which they are arranged ; C is the only exception.

It will be more satisfactory instead of treating the results separately as before, to discuss them in two groups, the first group containing subjects A, B, D, E, F ; the second group, C, G, H, and J.

Of the first group, A is the only one who omits card 1. The four dots on this card are very pale and undecided, just the kind of pink which the subject is apt to confuse with green. 2, 3, 7, 8, 15 and 16 are selected practically by all, the reds on these cards being either numerous or very bright. 10 and 14 seem not to be so easily recognized. The dots on 10 are mixed with blue or black and are impure. They may be mistaken for black by those of shortened spectrum, or be confused with the adjacent mole colour. 14 contains two contiguous fairly bright reds, a shade darker than those of card 1, but they were undiscriminated by A, B and D.

The cards wrongly inserted were 4, 6, 9, 12, 13 and particularly 11. Card 4 consists of green and grey dots only. The wrong insertion of card 4 is the mistake of A and F. The latter was the only one to insert 6 ; it consists of grey and green as before with yellowish-brown in addition. Card 11 has grey, sea-green and yellowish-brown dots ; 12 contains two very dark purples, which are generally mistaken for red. 13, chosen by F, confirmed his former choice of 4 and 6, for it is composed of greens and greys only. 9, which he includes, is a card of grey dots only.

These subjects all show confusion of reds, greens and greys. The test has many advantages, for it requires little apparatus and involves little time. It could be extended by asking the examinee to point to the red dots, and valuable information would be obtained as to the nature of the existing defect.

D was the only subject who made no mistakes, but then he only selected three cards out of a possible 9, which clearly points to defect of some kind. If results were based on this part alone of Nagel's test, he is the only one who would require further testing. It is evident, however, that some reds can be distinguished, for the correct cards cannot all be selected by chance.

The second group of subjects show entire failure to recognize the red cards, and those which they have selected are faulty, except in the case of G. H could find no suitable cards, for he saw all the pinks on the cards as blues.

2. Red Spots only

Correct	3			
A	3	8		
B	3			15
C	none			
D	none			
E	3			15
F	3		9	15
G	none			
H	none			
J	none			

No subject answered this second question correctly. Those who selected the proper card, added a second erroneous card. Card 8, selected by A, contained bright greens and moles ; 9 was all grey, and 15 had some greens. It is curious that F should choose the card as containing reds spots only which contains nothing but grey spots.

3. Green only

Correct	5														
A	none														
B	none														
C	3	5	7	8	9	10	15								
D	4	5	9												
E	5	12													
F	none														
G	1	2	3	4	5	6	9	10	11	12	13	14	15	16	
H	none														
J	7														

This test again is valuable for picking out the colour-blinds. Subject G's result is remarkable : he chooses 14 cards out of the 16 possible. There is here evidently a very big confusion of red and green, for the majority of the cards selected have vivid red spots on them. Number 15 was previously considered correct in answer to question 1. Subject C, too, chose quite a few cards. It is note-worthy that A and B failed in this part of the test ; D fared badly also.

4. Grey only

Correct   **9**

A	1
B	none
C	none
D	3
E	7 9
F	none
G	none
H	3 9
J	All 16 cards

J's result is noteworthy, but very characteristic. All 16 cards appear to him as shades of grey. This agrees with all our previous findings. A omitted card 1 when selecting cards containing red spots ; it is now selected, showing confusion of red with grey. Card 3 has red spots only.

This part of Nagel's test is most satisfactory, and detects all the subjects.

Section B

In this section the subjects are asked to name the colours on four different cards, containing variously-coloured dots. This part does not seem of such intrinsic value as the first portion, and appears unnecessary.

B 1

Correct :	*Dark Purple*	*Green*	*Chocolate-Brown*
A	Red	Brown	Brown
B	Red	Green	Green
C	dark Green	Brown	Brown
D	Brown	Green	dark Grey
E	dark Red	Greenish Brown	Brown
F	Red	Orange	Orange
G	Green	Green	very dark Green
H	dark Brown	dark Brown	light Brown
J	Black	medium Grey	medium Grey

These show for all the subjects typical results, such as have been obtained from previous tests. C shows confusion of the purple with green, and does not recognize the green. D does not discern the purple ; G sees all the dots as green.

B 2

Correct:	Bright Red	Chocolate-Brown	Dark Brown
A	Red	Reddish	Brown
B	Red	Green	Green
C	Red	Green	dark Green
D	Red	Brown	dark Grey
E	Red	dark Red	Brown
F	Brown	Red	Red
G	Red	Red	Red
H	dark Brown	light Brown	Brown
J	light Grey	light Grey	dark Grey

This card contains the bright reds, which some of the subjects can identify. The browns are confused with reds and greens.   Subject G saw all the spots as red and J all of them as grey.

B 3

Correct :	Dark Green	Medium Green	Grey
A	Green	Green	Green
B	Green	Green	Green
C	Green	Green	Green
D	Green	Green	Green
E	Green	light Green	Grey
F	Red	Brown	Grey or light Red
G	Green	Green	Green
H	Grey	Brown	Grey
J	medium Grey	medium Grey	light Grey

The results for this card are very similar, and show the general confusion of green and grey.

B 4

Correct:	Dark Brown	Chocolate-Brown	Bright Red
A	Red	Red	Red
B	Green or Brown	Green	Red
C	Green	light Brown	Red
D	Brown	Brown	Red
E	Brown	Brown	Red
F	Brown	Green	Red
G	Red	Green	Red
H	Brown	Grey	Brown
J	Majority Black ; some light Greys		

The bright red spots are recognized by subjects A to G. This particular red always seems to be correctly identified. A, however, sees all the dots as red. Brown is a difficult colour and is confused either with red or green.

This part of the test is not so satisfactory as part A. It does not yield additional data to any extent, except to show the prevalent confusion. Part A is much more instructive and valuable, and reveals immediately the presence of any colour anomaly. Undoubtedly, it is most reliable as a test for colour-blinds, and its use is to be commended.

10. *The Edridge-Green Lantern*

This lantern was devised to detect all dangerous colour-blinds, and is the result of much research and practical experience. " The lantern contains five discs ; three carrying seven coloured glasses, one carrying seven[1] different sized apertures and one obturator, and one carrying seven modifying glasses. Each disc has a clear aperture. The other mechanical details are :—An electric lamp holder in a parabolic reflector, handles for moving the discs, and the indicating ring showing the colour, aperture

[1] The lantern used only contained six apertures.

or modifier in use. The discs are numbered 1—5 on side plates under handles."[1]

Disc No. 1 contains the different sized apertures, the largest of which was used throughout the experiment. The size of the aperture is intended to correspond to the distance of the examinee from a 5½-inch railway signal lamp, or from a 7-inch ship's lamp. The distance of 20 feet from the largest aperture (0·75 inch) is equivalent to a distance of 50 yards from a railway signal, 40 feet away is equivalent to a distance of 100 yards, 80 feet away to a distance of 200 yards, and so on. As such distances may not be available in actual testing, the aperture may be reduced instead—one foot away from the smallest aperture equals a distance of 50 yards from the signal, 2 feet away 100 yards, etc. The lantern, therefore, is useful for detecting those cases in which red and green can be distinguished near at hand, but not at a distance. Such cases are certainly dangerous, and should be rejected for practical purposes.

The distance from the lantern during the tests was about 3 feet instead of 20—the reason being that the tests were not being applied for practical purposes, but merely to aid in an investigation of colour defect.

The second, third, and fourth discs contain the coloured glasses. In order they are as follows :—(1) clear, (2) red A, (3) red B, (4) yellow, (5) green, (6) signal-green, (7) blue, (8) purple. The three discs are similar in every respect. The colours are brought into view by moving one or more of the handles into position until they correspond with the scale at the top of the lantern. Edridge-Green has given a spectroscopic analysis of the light transmitted through each glass (*vide Colour-Blindness and Colour-Perception*). Red A is the signal red which presents

---

[1] Official description supplied with Lantern.

little difficulty to the colour-blind, but which is useful in combinations. Red B, a very decided red to the normal eye, is often mistaken for green by the colour-blind. Yellow is a most useful colour and is frequently misnamed. The pure green is troublesome, as is the signal-green also. The blue appears of a lavender shade, but, if desired, a purer blue is available by combining it with signal-green. The purple glass offers special features and aids in diagnosis.

Disc No. 5 contains the following modifying glasses :— (1) clear, (2) ground glass, (3) ribbed glass, (4) neutral 1, (5) neutral 2, (6) neutral 3, (7) neutral 4, (8) neutral 5.

The colour-blind can distinguish a difference between standard red and standard green close at hand in the same way that a normal person may be able to distinguish between a green and a blue-green. But if only one of these were to be shown, and particularly at a distance, with poor illumination its recognition would be impossible. In testing, therefore, it is necessary that the intensity of the light should be changed without the subject's know-ledge, and this is achieved by means of the neutral glasses, which modify the light so that it appears as it would under certain atmospheric conditions. The neutral glasses represent fog, the ground glass mist, and the ribbed glass rain. The normal-visioned can still distinguish the colours, except with the thickest neutral, but the colour-blind find the task a very difficult one.

The ground and ribbed glasses do not alter the colour of the light, but scatter it, and they diminish the lumin-osity of the whole of the spectrum. "The neutral glasses make the red appear like the green of the colour-blind and the green like the red."

No. 1 neutral diminishes the intensity of light.

No. 2 neutral imparts a faintly greenish light.

No. 3 neutral imparts an orange tinge.

No. 4 neutral imparts a reddish tinge.

No. 5 imparts a redder tinge.

The test is based on four principles :

(1) The colour-blind match colours according to their psycho-physical units. They actually judge by colour, and their judgments remain constant. The glasses employed in the lantern are those particularly liable to be confused by the colour-blind.

(2) The colour-blind name colours in accordance with their psycho-physical units and thus show to what class they belong. Guessing is improbable.

(3) Colours may be changed to the colour-blind, while remaining unaltered to the normal eye.

(4) Simultaneous contrast is more marked in the colour-blind than in the normal eye. A yellow contrasted with red appears green, and a yellow contrasted with green appears red—this is particularly characteristic of the three unit.

It will be noticed that in this test the candidate is asked to *name* the colours ; this is a striking feature of all Edridge-Green's tests. He believes, and rightly too, that if an examinee sees a red light, but says to himself, " That's green," then he is a source of danger to the community. By this test the colour-ignorant is excluded as well as the colour-blind ; the former can be re-examined at some later date if he so desires.

The candidate is to be rejected :

(1) If he calls the red green, or the green red, in any circumstances.

(2) If he calls the white light red, or green, or *vice versa*, in any circumstances.

(3) If he calls the red green, or the white light black, in any circumstances.

Any of these mistakes is sufficient evidence of defective

colour-vision ; if other mistakes are made the candidate requires a more thorough examination.

About twenty glasses in all are shown to each candidate, so that the test involves little time. It is advisable that it be conducted in a darkened room.

In the experiments conducted with the colour-blinds, seventy-six differently-coloured lights and combinations of light were tried with each subject, which gave a reliable estimate of the validity of the test. The light of the lantern was switched off after the subject had identified the colour, the handle readjusted, and then the light switched on again. It is important when two lights are being combined that the examinee does not see a green, for example, before it is altered by means of a modifying glass. This danger is removed when the handles are adjusted with the lantern's light extinguished. The experiment was conducted in a darkened room.

Below are given the glasses in the order in which they were shown. The subject was asked to name the colour visible to him.

1	Red A	19	Green + N. 4
2	Neutral 2	20	Red A + N. 4
3	Blue	21	Neutral 4
4	Purple + N. 4	22	N. 1 + Red B
5	Pure Green	23	Signal-Green
6	Neutral 3	24	Yellow + Pure Green
7	Blue + Signal-Green	25	Yellow + Pure Green + Purple
8	Clear	26	Neutral 5
9	Yellow + Blue	27	Neutral 1
10	Red B	28	Yellow
11	Ribbed Glass + Red B	29	Red A
12	Ground Glass	30	Yellow
13	Red A + Signal-Green	31	Green
14	Yellow	32	Yellow
15	Red B + Yellow + Signal-Green	33	Red A + N. 4
16	Ribbed Glass + Clear	34	Red A
17	Red A + Purple	35	Red A + N. 4
18	Purple	36	Yellow + Ground Glass

37	Red B+Pure Green	57	Yellow
38	Signal-Green+N. 5	58	Pure Green
39	Yellow+Ribbed Glass	59	Yellow
40	Blue+N. 4	60	Red B
41	Red A+Signal-Green+N. 3	61	Yellow
42	Yellow+N. 4	62	Green
43	Red B+Pure Green+N. 1	63	Red A
44	Purple+Yellow	64	Clear
45	Red B+Yellow+Pure Green	65	Red B
46	Red B+Pure Green+N. 2	66	Yellow
47	Red B+Signal-Green+Purple	67	Yellow+Yellow
48	Yellow+Pure Green+N. 4	68	Green
49	Green+Ground Glass	69	Green+Green
50	Blue+N. 3	70	Green
51	Pure Green+N. 5	71	Red B
52	Blue	72	Yellow
53	Signal-Green+Blue	73	Signal-Green
54	Blue	74	Purple
55	Purple	75	Blue
56	Pure Green	76	Purple+ N. 4

Red :

To make the results more comparable, the replies to red have been collected (including red A and red B, and combinations giving red). Red was shown twenty-seven times in all.

Recognized Red		*Confused*
A	20 times	Orange, 2 ; Green, 4 ; Colourless, 1.
B	16 ,,	Orange, 4 ; Green, 3 ; Yellow, 3 ; White, 1.
C	7 ,,	Green, 7 ; Grey, 3 ; Brown, 9 ; Colourless, 1.
D	24 ,,	Yellow, 1 ; Black, 1 ; White, 1.
E	20 ,,	Orange, 2 ; Grey, 1 ; Brown, 3 ; White, 1.
F	9 ,,	Brown, 6 ; Green, 2 ; Yellow, 2 ; Grey, 1 ; White, 1 ; Colourless, 2 ; Yellowish-Red, 4.
G	15 ,,	Green, 12.
H	0 ,,	Orange, 12 ; Yellow, 4 ; Black, 1 ; Grey, 9 ; White, 1.
J	0 ,,	White, 1 ; Black, 5 ; Grey, 20 ; Colourless, 1.

This Table shows the number of times red was recognized by each subject, and the number of confusions made with some other colour. H and J show complete failure in discriminating red, but the colours they mistake it for are not alike in each case. H saw it mainly as orange or yellow ; J, however, could perceive no colour, and all the glasses appeared as greys. There exists a common confusion of red with green, which is particularly notice-able in the case of G. This test gives good results with this subject ; he customarily tries to minimize his disability as far as possible, but the changes in the intensity of the light, with the insertion of modifying glasses, defeat his purpose.

If we analyse the responses further, we shall see more clearly the effects of the various modifying glasses.

Presented alone, red A was distinguished by A, B, D, E and G. C thought it was yellow or green, F yellow, H dark yellow, and J a dark grey. Combined with neutral 4 the colour became changed for C and G. Alone, G called it red ; shown with N. 4, which modifies the light so that it appears as in a thick fog, his judgment was changed to green.

Red B alone was recognized by A, B, C, D, E, and G. Combined with neutral 1, it remained unchanged for A, D, and G, but altered in colour for the others. For B it caused a change from red to yellow, for C, a change to light brown, for E a change to orange, and for F a change from yellowish-brown to yellowish-red. H and J, as before, saw the colours as orange and medium grey respectively, and they remained unaffected when com-bined with the modifier. Neutral 1 merely diminishes the intensity of light, but this was sufficient to cause a change of hue in the case of three of the subjects.

Edridge-Green recommends showing a colour with modifying glass, withdrawing the modifier, thus presenting the colour alone, and then replacing it. This was done with red A and neutral 4. The results were as follows :—

	Red A + N. 4	Red A	Red A + N. 4
A	Red	Red	Red
B	Red	Red or orange	Red
C	Green	light Brown	Green
D	Red	Red	Red
E	Red	light Red	dark Red
F	Yellowish Red	Yellowish Red	Red
G	Green	Red	Green
H	dark Grey	dark Yellow	dark Grey
J	Black	dark Grey	dark Grey

The effect of the neutral glass on subject G is clearly marked, for it completely changes the character of the light for him. It is interesting to note that the neutral glass causes a difference, too, in the case of subject H.

Green

The number of times green was correctly named was compiled in the same way. The numbers given include pure green, signal-green and combinations giving green. They will be analysed later. In all, green was presented 16 times.

	Recognized Green	Confused
A	9 times	Red, 1 ; Yellow, 6.
B	8 ,,	Orange, 3 ; Yellow, 2 ; Yellow-Green, 1 ; Red-Green 1 ; Black, 1.
C	2 ,,	Red, 1 ; Yellow, 2 ; Blue, 1 ; Brown, 3 ; White, 1 ; Grey, 5 ; just sees disc 1.
D	12 ,,	Red, 2 ; Yellow-Green, 1 ; Black, 1.
E	10 ,,	Brown, 2 ; Grey, 4.
F	0 ,,	Red, 5 ; Yellow, 2 ; Yellow-Red, 1 ; Black, 1 ; just sees disc 7.
G	13 ,,	Red, 1 ; Yellow-Red, 2.
H	0 ,,	Orange, 9 ; Yellow, 2 ; White, 1 ; Grey, 3 ; Black, 1.
J	0 ,,	Orange, 1 ; Grey, 13 ; Black, 2.

About half the number of greens shown was recognized by the better subjects. F, H, and J failed completely to recognize the colour. The green was more apt to be confused with orange and yellow than with red except in the case of F. It was surprising the number of times it was identified with a grey.

The results of pure and signal-green differed with the varying subjects ; they also differed when combined with neutral glasses.

	Green	Signal-Green	Green+N. 4	Sig.-Green+N. 5
A	Green	almost White	Green	Green
B	Yellow	Green	Green	Green
C	?	White	Blue	Grey
D	very light Green	very light Green	dark Green	Nothing
E	bright Green	light Green	Grey Brown	Grey
F	Yellow	pale Red	dark Red	Nothing
G	Green	Blue-Green	very dark Green	very dark Green
H	Yellow	White	dark Grey	dark Grey
J	very light Grey	very light Grey	very dark Grey	Black

The responses to the first two columns show differences for the same subject. A, for example, did not recognize signal-green, although discriminating pure green, and saw it as almost white. This would at once cause rejection if she were being tested for practical purposes. The lantern seems to detect the less severe cases of colourblindness as well as the extreme cases. C also saw this colour as white ; F showed confusion of it with red. B, although recognizing signal-green, failed to discriminate the pure green from yellow.

The neutral glasses with these colours did not trouble subject G as they did with the red, but that is no evidence of unreliability, for, if in doubt, he invariably ventured green.

The pure green disc was shown alone, then combined with the second green disc, which was afterwards withdrawn.

N

	Green	*Green + Green*	*Green*
A	Yellow	Green	Yellow
B	Green	Green	Yellow
C	Grey	Grey	Yellow or Grey
D	dark Green	Blue or Green	Green
E	Green	dark Green	light Green
F	Yellowish Brown	Yellowish Red	Yellowish Brown
G	Green	Green	Green
H	light Orange	dark Orange	light Orange
J	medium Grey	medium Grey	light Grey

With some, this change in intensity caused the colour to assume a deeper shade ; with others, it effected a complete change of hue. A was unable to identify the green alone, but combined with a second disc, the colour became recognizable. B was unaffected by the double disc, but by contrast the following single disc was changed in colour. The two discs in the case of F were sufficient to alter the judgment from a yellowish brown to a yellowish red.

Red A, combined with signal-green, appears a foggy red to the normal eye. This yielded interesting results. To A it appeared colourless ; to B a green. C, D, E, and H could see nothing ; and all that F and J could discern were grey and black respectively. G, curiously enough, was the only one who named the colour correctly. This is a most searching combination of discs, and laid bare each subject's defect.

Red B, combined with pure green, produces a yellow inclining to red. F saw it as a light red, and D as a yellowish white. To the other subjects it appeared green, except to J, who perceived it as a grey.

Yellow :

The yellow disc, of a deep orange colour, is a very useful one, and can be used alone or in combinations. It was presented 18 times.

Recognized Yellow		*Confused*
A	10 times	Orange, 3 ; Red, 2 ; Green, 2 ; Yellow-Green, 1.
B	3 ,,	Orange, 7 ; Red, 5 ; Green, 1 ; White, 2.
C	4 ,,	Red, 1 ; Green, 4 ; Brown, 9.
D	12 ,,	White, 1 ; Brown, 3 ; Yellow-Red, 1 ; White-Red, 1.
E	0 ,,	Orange, 5 ; Red, 2 ; Green, 2 ; White, 2 ; Brown, 7.
F	6 ,,	Red, 2 ; White, 2 ; Brown, 8.
G	1 ,,	Orange, 1 ; Red, 13 ; Green, 3.
H	5 ,,	Orange, 13.
J	0 ,,	Orange, 4 ; White, 1 ; Grey, 13.

The yellow was not always recognized as such ; although its frequent identification with orange may be considered permissible. Its constant confusion with red and green is more serious. Subject G thought it to be red 13 times, and green 3 times, and only recognized it correctly twice. C called it brown 9 times, E 7, and F 8 times, which is not a grave error. J gave his usual characteristic result for practically every time it appeared to him as grey. This confirms our previous findings of a reduced sensitivity to yellow.

If we take the results separately—for the above Table by collating results passes over many interesting facts— we find varied responses. The yellow disc alone was mistaken by B and G for red. Combined with N.4 (which changed the colour to red for the normal eye) it remained unchanged for B, but appeared green to G. The modifying glasses, as we have pointed out above, markedly affect colours for this subject. A, E, and F called the yellow orange ; combined with the neutral glass it became green for A, remaining unchanged for the others. C, D, and F named it brown ; with the modifying glass C saw it as a grey, D as red (correct) and F as green.

Showing the disc alone and then combining it with a second disc of yellow, left the colour unchanged for all the examinees except E, who called the double disc red in distinction to his previous designation of the single disc as orange.

Simultaneous and successive contrast is more marked in the colour-blind than in the normal-visioned. This is clearly shown by using a yellow, a red, and a green disc. To the normal eye, the yellow alters little when contrasted with the red or the green. To the colour-blind, however, the yellow may appear green when contrasted with a red, and red when contrasted with a green. This can be demonstrated with the Edridge-Green Lantern, and, as already noted, is one of the principles on which the lantern is based. Discs were shown in the order, yellow, red A, yellow, green, yellow. The only contrast effect with this sequence was with G, who called the yellow disc appearing after the red one, green.

A second set with the discs presented as follows, pure green, yellow, pure green, yellow, red B, yellow, green, red A, gave better results.

	Green	Yellow	Green	Yellow	Red B	Yellow	Green	Red A
A	Green	Yellow	Yellow	Yellow	Orange	Yellow	Yellow	Red
B	Orange	Red	Red-Green	Orange	not Red but Red-Orange	Red-Orange	Green	Orange
C	Green	light Brown	light Brown	light Brown	light Brown	light Brown	light Brown	Red
D	Green-Yellow	Yellow	Green	Yellow	dark Red	Yellow	light Green	Red
E	light Brown	Orange	Green	Orange	Red	Brown	Green	Red
F	Yellow-Brown	Yellow-Brown	Yellow-Brown	Yellow-Brown	Yellow-Brown	Yellow-Brown	Yellow-Brown	Yellow-Red
G	Yellow-Red	Red	Green	Orange	Red	Red	Green	Red
H	Orange	dark Orange	dark Orange	v. dark Orange	v. v. d. Orange	Orange	light Orange	v. dark Orange
J	light Grey	Orange	medium Grey	Orange	dark Grey	medium Grey	medium Grey	dark Grey

The effect of contrast is clear in certain cases ; the yellow is called green or it is seen as red. Occasionally the yellow affects the green or the red following. Very often the green appears yellow when it has been preceded by that colour. Note that B describes yellow as red, and the green which follows it he designates as reddish green. Subject G, as before, has heightened contrast and his yellows are changed according to the previous colours. With H and J it is interesting to observe that the contrast effect takes the form of a difference in shade.

Yellow and pure green combined appear a yellowish green to the normal eye. This was seen as green by A, B, D, and E, yellow by C, yellowish brown by F, orange by H and J, and red by G.

Blue :

The blue disc was presented twice only. It is not a pure blue, but appears of a lavender shade. All subjects identified it with blue, however, except A, who once called it violet, and D, who described it as blue+red. A pure blue is obtained by combining the blue disc with signal-green. The subjects experienced no difficulty in recognizing the pure colour, although D was doubtful as to whether it was a green or a blue. This indicates that blue is a clear sensation to them, that is one of their best colours. The " three-unit " of Edridge-Green who see green, red and violet, have difficulty with blues, which seems peculiar, for repeatedly the colour-blinds are able to recognize this colour better than any other. They certainly cannot distinguish blue from violet or purple, but this confusion stands in a totally different category from the mistakes made with reds and greens.

Blue combined with N.3 or N.4 produces a rose colour. This was correctly indicated by five of the subjects.

C named it red with N.3, but grey with N.4; G both times identified it with green ; H and J saw both as greys.

Purple :

This disc was shown alone three times and to most subjects it appeared a blue. B always qualified his answer, and stated it was a different blue from the others. This shows he was able to detect some difference between it and the blue or violet disc. H and J discerned it quite readily as blue, which is so different from J's usual series of greys. E described it once as blue and red, once as purple and red, and once as red with a purple edge. He never seemed to see the disc all one colour. D named it dark green, blue and red, and dark red respectively.

Purple combined with N.4 yields a sensation of red. It was correctly named by A, B, D, and G. C saw it as brown ; E recognized it the first time, but the second time he described it as " dark with orange in it." F with difficulty could just discern the disc. To H and J it appeared grey.

Neutrals :

The neutrals were shown alone as single glasses. There are five in all : the colours they gave to the light is shown in brackets.

The light itself was seen as a greenish yellow by A and a green by C. The other subjects all saw it as a white light. (See page 167.)

These columns show the difference that a modifier makes to the light of the lantern. N.3, N.4, and N.5 change the light from red to green for A. With B the light remains unaltered and the red effect which is very plain to normal vision has no existence for him. C manifests great confusion of green with red, and the neutrals effectively

	N. 1 (*Yellow*)	N. 2 (*Yellow*)	N. 3 (*Orange*)	N. 4 (*Red*)	N. 5 (*Red*)
A	Yellow	almost Yellow	Green	Green	Green
B	pale Yellow	Yellow	Yellow	Yellow	Orange
C	Yellow	Green	Crimson	Green	light Brown
D	Yellow-White	Red	White-Yellow-Red	Red	Red
E	light Brown	Red	Brown	Red with Yellow	Red
F	Yellow	pale Yellow	Reddish-Yellow	Green	Green
G	Red	Red	Red	Red	Green
H	dark Yellow	light Yellow	dark Yellow	Orange	dark Orange
J	medium Grey	light Grey	dark Grey	medium Grey	very dark Grey

change the light in a most erratic manner. E exhibits confusion with Neutrals 1 and 3. N.4 and N.5 trouble subject F, and change the light from red to green. G has difficulty with N.1 and N.2, and N.5 causes a complete change of judgment. The effect on H is to darken the light. J, as before, remains impervious to all changes.

These results speak well for the value of the neutral glasses, and support Edridge-Green's dictum that they " make red appear like the green of the colour-blind, and the green like the red." They make a very effective test, and show how greatly atmospheric conditions alter the colour of a light to the colour-blind. They seem to pick out the weak points immediately, and have clearly manifested the fact that all the subjects are " dangerous " colour-blinds. As forming part of an excellent practical test, they are thoroughly to be relied upon.

Ground Glass:

With the ground glass the light appeared white to most of the subjects. A, however, described it as " red, with more yellow in it." For C it changed the light to a green, and to G a faint yellow-green was visible.

G found the ground glass troublesome, and it took him always a considerable time to decide on the colours when so modified. It did not affect the other subjects so much. In front of the yellow glass, it changed the colour for G to red. In front of the green glass, it altered the colour to a yellow-red, which he found most difficult to distinguish. The only other result was to transform the green glass to an orange in B's case.

The ground glass does not appear to be effective with all colour-blinds, but in some cases it may completely alter the colour of the light.

Ribbed Glass:

The ribbed glass in front of the light produced no change in colour except with subject C. In his case it altered the light to green. In front of red B, it had no effect on any of the subjects, the red merely appearing to them as it did without the modifying glass. Combined with the yellow light, it resulted in no change of judgment. G called the colour red, but he described the light alone as red, so that the ribbed glass produced no alteration. This glass, apparently, does not seem to be of much utility, at least if these results are reliable.

Combination of Colours:

It is very useful in testing to combine colours. Certain discs presented together produce black, which is useful in cases of shortened spectrum. If a black were never shown, a colour-blind would hesitate to call any combination of discs black.

Red A + Signal-Green + N.3.
Red B + Pure Green + Purple.
Yellow + Pure Green + Purple.

These three combinations were included in the test at irregular intervals. They were all described as black by the subjects.

Yellow + pure green + N.4 is also a valuable combination. It appears as a whitish grey. Some colour-blinds call it green, others red, and some are just able to see the disc.

Edridge-Green advocates in any examination the presentation of a red made from red A and purple. This gave informative results.

Red A + Purple (*Red*)

A   Red
B   Red
C   Green
D   Red
E   dark Red
F   See light only
G   dark Green
H   dark Grey
J   Black

This is a very useful red to show. It may be confused with green, or, in cases of a shortened spectrum, it may appear a black. This is the reason why it is advisable to combine colours such as we described above, to produce sensations of black.

Yellow in conjunction with purple forms another red which is useful for diagnostic purposes. In this test it was discriminated by subjects A—F. G described it as green, however, and H and J as a very dark grey.

Three other combinations are worthy of mention for the results they yield.

Red B + Yellow + Signal-Green = Red (1).

Red B + Yellow + Pure Green = Red (2).

Red B + Pure Green + N 3 = Green (3).

	(1) Red	(2) Red	(3) Green
A	Red	Red	Green
B	Green	Green	Black
C	Brown or Green	Grey	Grey
D	Dirty Red	light Yellow	Red
E	Grey Brown	Grey Brown	Steel Grey
F	Red	Red	Red
G	Green	dark Green	Green
H	dark Grey	dark Grey	Black
J	Black	very dark Grey	Nothing

It will be seen from the Table above that these three combinations are highly instructive. A is the only subject who names the colours correctly. The others reveal confusion from B downwards, even D showing complete inability to discriminate the colours. This is an example of the many combinations of discs which can be produced by this lantern, and which aid in making it so satisfactory a test.

Aperture 3 :

The above experiments were all carried out using the large aperture. Only one or two of the subjects were tried with Aperture 3.

For C it changed red A to yellow, and made all the other colours appear white ; even blue was reduced to a grey.

E merely saw each colour (red A, red B, yellow, green, signal-green) as a spot of light. He recognized the blue and saw the purple as a darker shade.

To F red A remained unaltered : red B appeared orange : yellow and pure green were discriminated, the former called brown; thus he retained his former terminology. Signal-green, however, was seen as a dark grey, which is a significant mistake.

The lantern test as a whole is most comprehensive,

and proved very reliable. The subjects tested by it are all diagnosed as " dangerous " colour-blinds. It has the advantage that the results obtained from one lantern are constant and therefore comparable with one another. The colours used are precisely those which are most confused by the colour-blinds. The lantern is easy to work, and so many combinations can be made and the order of testing can be changed so frequently, that no coaching will enable a colour-blind to elude detection. This avoids the criticism urged against so many otherwise excellent tests. For practical purposes it has the great advantage that the effect of atmospheric conditions on colours is tested, and we have seen how misleading that effect can be when it is a question of colour-blindness.

Undoubtedly, this test is one of the best which has yet been evolved. It is based on the actual sensations which the colour-blind experience, and the recognition of colours, which is to so great an extent the basis of the method of testing, is, in itself, of supreme importance. The test combines the advantages of showing " confusion " colours with the naming of colours, and avoids all the defects which usually make tests involving nomenclature so unreliable and untrustworthy. It is a test to be highly commended.

11. *Painting Test*

(a) *Coloured Diagrams*

For this test I am indebted to Professor Roaf, of Cardiff, who has kindly allowed me to make use of this test here. He is working out a test on a new principle, and subjects the paintings to a spectral analysis. The paintings consist of squares divided geometrically into 25 parts, each differently coloured, with the colours in some cases repeated twice. A special box of paints containing 15 pigments is used throughout—no mixing of paints is necessary, and the examinee is allowed to try the paints on a spare piece of paper first.[1]

Professor Roaf's scheme is not so much a test for colour-blindness as a new attempt to analyse cases, to find out by a simple method what part of the spectrum is defective.

The pigments being impure reflect a fairly wide region of the spectrum. If an individual fails to appreciate one part of the spectrum as different from another part he may do one of three things. He may match colours correctly either by accident, or by shade, or some other means. He may add the colour which he does not recognize or he may subtract that colour. If he fails to recognize red he may add red to green, thus putting a yellow, grey, or some such colour to match green. He may subtract red from grey or yellow, putting green as a match for the neutral colours, or match blue and purple. If the mistakes all occur in one region of the spectrum, the colour-blind's copy and the original can be matched by examining them in light deficient in the rays in which the colour-blind differs from the normal.

The paintings are examined through colour screens and in the recombined spectrum after certain parts of the spectrum have been cut out. Colour screens are used and different regions of the spectrum are cut out, until the abnormal painting matches the original. This is possible, exclusive of slight differences of shade. When the minimum amount of reduction possible to give an

[1] See *Journal of Physiology*, vol. LVII ; and *Quarterly Journal of Experimental Physiology*, nos. 1 and 2, 1924 : Articles by Professor Roaf.

absolute match is made, the region of the spectrum defective for that individual can be ascertained.

The paintings determine, therefore, the wave-length of light that the individual colour-blind person fails to recognize as different in a particular region of the spectrum.

The paintings done by three of the subjects tested are appended. (See Figure VII.)[1] They are not given in their original colours, but have been redrawn in black and white. They lose considerably in the transference, and the results of all the subjects have not been included. A description, however, of the paintings of all the subjects tested throws light upon the diagram from a psychological point of view.

Apart from the spectral analysis which the paintings reveal, they are interesting also for themselves alone, and the errors committed by the colour-blind are illuminative of their defect.

A. Started with blues, then yellows. The painting exhibits the customary confusion of blues with violets ; the pale lavender is mistaken for pale blue. The pale green is painted pale lavender at one time, but pale blue takes its place at another time. The red is correctly matched as is also the magenta, but much hesitation is displayed in the greens. The jade green appears a grey, which the subject thought was a blue-green. (This is the subject's neutral band.) The two browns cause trouble ; they are both represented by vivid green. The orange is not distinguished from light brown.

B. Started, as in the case above, with blues and yellows. His efforts show confusion of blues and purples. He found the test difficult, but matched the colours with wonderful

---

[1] These are from copies, the originals of which are in the possession of Professor Roaf.

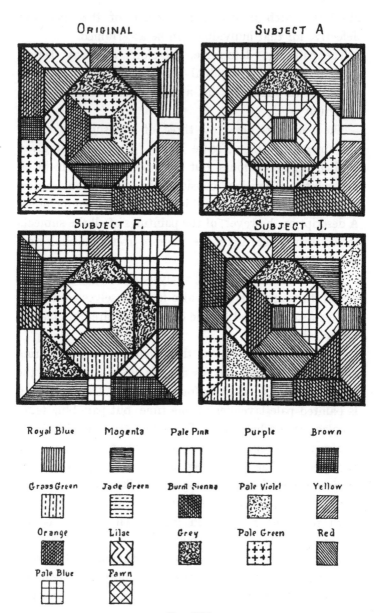

Fig. VII.

accuracy ; and produced a fair copy of the original. For pale green, he tried dark green, magenta, pale green, then gave it up, but ultimately returned to pale green. The pale pink is represented by grey on both occasions. The green is correctly matched, but the grey is represented by a vivid green. The red and magenta are correctly matched.

C. Found the test very difficult. His reproduction of the pigments is remarkable for the pale shades he used. Probably the pale colours are a sign of additional confusion, and Professor Roaf concurs in this opinion. This effort displays poor colour-perception, for yellow is practically the only colour properly matched. The blue and purple on the outside of the diagram are correct, but in the centre the purple (dark and pale) is mistaken for blue. The reds are not recognized, but are matched with orange, probably thought to be brown. This is the form of confusion which red generally takes with this subject. On the magenta triangle, he tried pink first of all, then washed it out, tried green, and finally brown. Pink is represented by grey at one time, and by very pale green at another. The greens are differently matched ; the bright or grass green is replaced by pink, the pale greens by pale pink. The jade green is matched with grey and *vice versa*. The pale shades, such as the lavenders and very pale blues, do not seem to have been recognized at all, and must have appeared colourless to the subject. The browns, too, are not discriminated from the burnt sienna. This whole painting reveals faulty matching, and points to the defect being of a grave nature. This confirms all the results obtained from this subject except those from the colour equations.

E. E began with yellows, and found most difficulty with the pale colours, grey, green, and pink. The diagram is very correctly matched, and only the following errors are made : blue and violet, pale green and pale blue.

F. Experienced great difficulty in selecting the colours to match. This reproduction contains a large number of confusions. The yellow is the only colour which is painted correctly. The blues and violets are interchanged. The lavenders are represented by a pale blue in one case, and a pale green in the other. The reds and magentas show a curious mixture. The red is represented correctly at one time, but is matched with magenta elsewhere. The magenta, however, is not distinguished from blue. This corresponds with the confusion-skeins chosen in matching the magenta skein in the Holmgren wool test. The pale pinks are mistaken for greys. The greens are variously represented. Grass green is shown by a fawn colour, jade green by magenta. Between this latter and the red no distinction is made, but they are both painted indiscriminately the same colour ; plainly, they must have appeared similar in hue to the subject. The pale greens are matched with pale pinks. The browns, too, show confusion, in one place with green, in another with orange. One part of the diagram appeared unpainted to the subject.

G. This subject, as indicated before, is a difficult one to test, as he is always endeavouring to cover his defect, and employs as many artifices as he can devise. The painting test was no exception. He tried out a great number of colours to begin with on the spare paper, and decided there were not enough colours in the box. The blues were too blue or not blue enough. (*N.B.*—The confusion between the blues and the purples—he saw no difference in the two adjoining colours on the outside of the diagram, but painted them all a uniform purple.) He held the spare paper close to the coloured diagram, each time trying different colours, until he found one which gave a satisfactory match ; it was not till then that he painted in the colour on the allotted space.

The greens he left to the end, simply because he could not match them—he ultimately painted them correctly but by the merest chance. For magenta he resorted to trying out all the colours still dry ! His diagram is wonderfully accurate, the only confusion being lavender with green and pink with grey.

This painting is a good example of the resources of an educated subject aware of his defect.

H. H took 1¼ hours to paint his diagram, a much longer time than any of the others. He found the colours very difficult to match and, like G, tried a large number of them before deciding on the correct one. With pink, for example, he had no idea what colour it was, nor with what colour he was matching it, and he went entirely by shade. A slight difference in shade was a big factor in the ultimate decision, so that dilution of the pigment played a large part in the matches made. This is evident in the fact that the same colour is sometimes differently matched.

It will be noticed that the magentas are correctly represented. The reds, however, show confusion, and in one case red is matched with brown. The jade green is accurately painted, but the same green is used as a match for brown, showing that the former correct match is probably accidental. The grass green is mistaken for light brown.

The pale colours reveal perplexity. Pink is matched correctly in one case, but is confused in another case with grey. Lavender and pale greens are interchanged. Blues and purples are not distinguished, and the orange is not differentiated from the burnt sienna.

J. Started with yellows and blues. He matched the jade green by mere accident, for on questioning the subject

o

after he had completed the painting, it was found that pink also was considered a good match. He chose colours by their brightness value only. Red, which is in the right place, he thought was black. Magenta was the most difficult of all ; he saw it as an impure black, which he matched correctly by the chance device of going over all the colours in the paint-box until he found one of the same shade.

It was very noticeable with this subject that when he started to fill in part of the diagram and went back to the box for more paint, he often forgot what colour he had been using, and sometimes had to begin all over again.

The diagram itself shows confusion of blue with purple ; red with brown ; pink with lavender. The grass green is matched with orange, and the jade green with a pale shade of the grass green.

These paintings give typical results and show the confusions which exist with colour-blinds. From the observations made during the painting, one fact stands out clearly, that shade is a potent factor. A difference in shade which means no alteration of colour for normal vision, effects a change in hue for the colour-blind. It is noteworthy, too, that yellow and blue were the first colours to be matched by the majority of the subjects.

Professor Roaf, who submitted the original drawings to a spectral analysis, very kindly sent me the results he obtained.

The results show what wave-lengths must be excluded from the spectrum of an arc lamp in order that the copy and the original may match. There are three Tables:—

(1) Of progressive cutting off of the red end of the spectrum.

(2) Of viewing the diagrams in a limited region of the spectrum.

(3) Of cutting out a band in the spectrum.

+ means that the diagram matches the original.

— means that it does not match.

? means that it almost matches, but that there may exist a difference in colour that would be recognized by an independent observer.

o means that no observation was made.

The results are appended without comment.

Table 1

	6629	6552	6353	6346	6202	6128	6002	5926	5827	5625	5222	4973
A	o	o	—	o	o	—	—	—	—	+	o	o
B	o	o	—	o	o	—	—	?	?	?	?	+
C	o	o	o	o	o	o	—	o	—	o	o	o
E	—	—	+	+	+	+	o	o	o	o	o	o
F	o	o	—	o	o	—	—	—	—	?	—	?
G	—	—	?	+	+	+	o	o	o	o	o	o
H	o	o	—	o	o	—	—	?	?	+	o	o
J	o	o	—	o	o	—	—	—	—	?	+	o

Table 2

	6346–5827	6031–5625	5096–4844	4946–4733	4733–4165
A	—	?	+	—	+
B	+	+	+	+	+
C	o	o	o	o	o
E	+	+	+	+	+
F	—	?	?	—	+
G	+	+	+	+	+
H	—	?	?	—	+
J	—	—	—	—	+

Table 3

	6779–5827	6779–4953	6678–6377	6678–6346	6678–6202	6678–6002	6678–5852	6678–5726	6678–5648
A	—	—	o	o	—	—	—	—	?
B	—	—	o	o	—	—	?	?	?
C	—	—	o	o	—	—	—	—	+
E	+	o	—	+	+	+	+	+	+
F	—	—	o	o	—	—	—	—	?
G	+	o	—	+	+	+	+	+	+
H	—	—	o	o	—	—	?	?	?
J	—	—	o	o	—	—	—	—	?

Table 3

(*continued*)

	6527–4872	6527–4893	6580–6101	6402–5775	6429–5978	6377–4844
A	—	o	o	o	o	o
B	?	o	o	o	o	o
C	o	o	o	o	o	o
E	+	—	?	?	?	—
F	—	o	o	o	o	o
G	—	—	?	?	?	—
H	—	o	o	o	o	o
J	—	o	o	o	o	o

(*continued*)

	6353–6202	6353–5978	6353–5799	6127–5954	6328–4795
A	o	o	o	—	—
B	o	o	o	—	—
C	o	o	o	o	—
E	—	—	—	—	—
F	o	o	o	—	—
G	—	—	—	—	—
H	o	o	o	—	—
J	o	o	o	—	—

Professor Roaf finds that his subjects can be divided into three groups : (a) when the red end of the spectrum is cut off up to λ 6200. These show only one mistake, the confusion of blue with purple. This is explained by a shortening of the spectrum, *i.e.* an absolute lack of stimulation by a portion of the extreme red end of the spectrum. The conclusion is that such subjects " seem to recognize some differential effect of the spectrum between λ 5800 and the extreme red end of the spectrum, but they do not have as great a discrimination for red as a normal person."[1]

(b) The second group matches when the spectrum is cut off as far as γ 5800. In this group other confusions are made in addition to blue and purple ; for example,

[1] *Loc. cit.*, p. 155.

green and grey. The diagrams cannot be matched if the least trace of the red end of the spectrum is present.

(c) The third group requires the spectrum to be cut off to about λ 4800, leaving only the violet end of the spectrum in which to view the colours. In this class the diagrams show confusion of red and green. They will not match if any of the red end of the spectrum is present, nor if any of the green region is in the recombined light. They match when the spectrum is cut off to λ 4800. They show one peculiarity not shown by the other two groups. If they are examined in light from a narrow region of the spectrum, so that a monochromatic effect is produced, they will match in light from the yellow region from about λ 5500 to λ 6000, depending on the width of the band used.[1]

These results have led Professor Roaf to a hypothesis which was first formulated by Schultze in 1866.[2] To quote from the same article, Roaf states that " In studying the coloured globules in the retinæ of birds he (Schultze) pointed out that any light reaching the cones must be filtered through the corresponding globules, hence any light that is perceived must be that which can pass through the globules in front of the cone. In other words, the colour perception by a cone depends upon the filter placed in front of it, and the photo-chemical processes by which the nerve impulse is produced may be the same in all cones. This colour-filter hypothesis, which is comparable to the result produced by a Lumière or Paget plate negative, can explain most if not all the phenomena of colour vision.

. . . . " This aspect of the subject is being investigated. For instance, in a preliminary examination of

---

[1] *Loc. cit.*, p. 156.
[2] *Arch. f. mikr. Anat.*, I, 1866, p. 255.

the retina of a hen it was found that the red globules cut off daylight to about λ 5800, whilst the yellow globules cut off the spectrum to about λ 5000."[1]

Professor Roaf concludes : " It is premature to discuss this subject in detail, but I hope to pursue the investigation and test its application to colour-vision in man."[1]

(b) Coloured Picture

The copying of coloured pictures by colour-blinds forms a most instructive test.   The painting (original and copy) shown in the frontispiece is one executed by subject J, and is submitted as a point of further interest.   A number of such paintings would make an intensely fascinating collection.   The original painting was placed before the subject, along with an outline of the object shown, and he was instructed to copy the colours of the original.   Only six pigments were given, red, green, blue, yellow, pink, and brown.   Although the limited number of the colours may seem to suggest less confusion, and perhaps offer a little guidance to the colour-blind, such does not seem to have been the result.   With all the subjects tested, the characteristic confusions made themselves evident.

The reproduction in the frontispiece is a typical example of J's work along these lines.   His paintings exhibit a general but regular confusion.   Red and green are inter-changed promiscuously ;   yellow is confused with green, and pink with blue.   It will be noticed that, in the picture, the blue sky is represented by pink, and the green sea by brown.   The red splash at the side is an interesting feature.   The red was judged to be too dark to represent the beach—so green was substituted, as it was of a lighter shade of the *same* colour, and in consequence gave a more satisfactory match with the original.

[1] *Loc. cit.*, p. 158.

12. *Colour Preference*

A test of colour preference was carried out by the subjects themselves by the method of paired comparison, and I was able to obtain the results for some of them. The colours were six in number, magenta, red, blue, green, yellow, and violet ; and they were presented in pairs— the subject each time indicating the colour preferred. There were thirty pairs in all, which were arranged in chance order, involving thirty judgments. The experiment was so arranged that fatigue would be avoided, ten judgments only being made at one stretch ; the colours arranged by the experimenter were kept hidden until a given signal by means of a cover sheet. The same area of colour was shown in each case, the two colours being slipped into a specially devised apparatus somewhat resembling a double photograph frame. The whole experiment was regulated by means of a metronome.

	Magenta	*Red*	*Blue*	*Green*	*Yellow*	*Violet*
A	4	2	10	0	9	5
B	6	4	10	3	0	7
D	1	8	9	1	6	5
H	2	2	13	0	8	5

B thought the magenta was purple, and the violet blue. H thought likewise, but he also considered the red to be brown and the green grey.

In all four cases, green is more or less disliked, and is only chosen four times out of a possible 120—red also in the case of A, B, and H.

Blue and violet combined give the following results :—

A chose them 15 times
B   ,,   ,, 17 ,,
D   ,,   ,, 14 ,,
H   ,,   ,, 18 ,,

and together they form half the choice. The violet in many cases was thought to be blue.

$$
\text{Blue}+\text{Violet}+\text{Yellow} \begin{cases} \text{A} & - & 24 \text{ times out of } 30 \\ \text{B} & - & 17 \text{ ,,} \quad\quad \text{,,} \quad 30 \\ \text{D} & - & 20 \text{ ,,} \quad\quad \text{,,} \quad 30 \\ \text{H} & - & 24 \text{ ,,} \quad\quad \text{,,} \quad 30 \end{cases}
$$

This seems to point to the fact that the easily distinguished colours are the favourite ones, and those difficult to see are generally disliked.

It will be advisable to follow Professor Hayes' plan and gather together on a single page the results of all the experiments ; that is in so far as red or green was able to be distinguished. Red indicates that red was recognized with fair frequency in the test, Green that green was recognized. " Confusion " indicates that the typical colour-blind confusions took place. It can be clearly seen from the evidence that the subjects are not all limiting cases, and that red and green can be seen by some red-green colour-blinds.

	A	B	C	D	E	F	G	H	I	J
Stilling Test	red	red	confusion	red green	confusion	confusion	confusion	confusion	confusion	confusion
Holmgren Wools	confusion	confusion	confusion	red	confusion	confusion	confusion	confusion	confusion	confusion
Nomenclature	red green	red green	confusion	red green	red green	red green	red green	confusion	confusion	confusion
Colour-mixing	red	red	red green	red green	red	red green	red	confusion	confusion	confusion
Rayleigh Equation ...	red green	red green	red	green	green	red green	red	confusion	—	confusion
Colour Shadows	red	red green	confusion	green	red green	red	confusion	confusion	—	confusion
Colour Contrasts	red	red green	confusion	confusion	green	red	confusion	confusion	—	confusion
After-Images	red	red green	confusion	red green	confusion	confusion	confusion	confusion	—	confusion
Bradley Test	red	red	confusion	red green	red	confusion	red	confusion	—	confusion
E.G. Lantern	confusion	confusion	confusion	red green?	red green	confusion	confusion	confusion	—	confusion
Nagel Cards............	red?	red?	confusion	confusion	confusion	confusion	confusion	confusion	—	confusion
Painting Test	red	green	confusion	—	red green	confusion	red?green?	confusion	—	confusion

The number of times red and green can be distinguished relative to the number of confusions, gives a fair indication of the degree of the defect. H and J failed completely in every test, and may be regarded as limiting cases.

The Tests

All the tests used yielded satisfactory results. The most unsatisfactory are what may be termed the subjective tests, those tests over which no objective control is possible. The most marked are the after-images and the contrast experiments. In the former, it is difficult to regulate the time of perceiving the stimulus, for it was found sometimes that an after-image made its appearance with prolonged fixation where no image had been previously reported. The rings contrast, too, are unreliable. The coloured shadow is a better test, but varies with different experimenters unless an analysis of the source of light is possible. Colour equations, though trustworthy with reliable subjects, are not altogether satisfactory, for the experimenter is entirely dependent on the subjects and has no control over the final equation.

Tests involving comparison seem preferable, in which the examinee is asked to do something himself. Holmgren's Wool Test in its original or in a modified form holds the field here. Although discredited from time to time, chiefly because of its implication of the Young-Helmholtz theory, it has remained one of the best simple modes of testing. The improvements have taken two forms: (1) either the number of confusion colours has been reduced, or (2) the test skeins have been altered. The principle of the test, however, has remained unchanged. The Bradley Paper Test is devised somewhat along the same lines, but in addition it has the advantage that it gives a fairly reliable spectral analysis where more exact methods are not available.

Stilling's Tables and the Nagel Card Test also deserve commendation, for they have both been found to be excellent for testing purposes. They are useful for detecting the presence of an abnormality, but for diagnosis they require supplementing. Part B of Nagel's test does not seem to be of much service, and could be dispensed with. Part A forms an admirable test.

The Edridge-Green lantern is a test in a category by itself. It proved to be a most efficient one in every way. It has been devised after a long period spent in practical work with the colour-blinds, and is based on a thorough knowledge of their characteristics. For practical purposes it should prove of the very highest value. It combines the recognition of colours with the naming of them, which was found to be of great utility throughout the experiments. The modifying glasses are well adapted for the purposes intended, and proved most satisfactory. The test has the advantage that a short examination with it is sufficient to reveal the defect. Further, it seems impossible to coach a colour-blind to pass such a test, so many combinations of glasses are possible.

CHAPTER VI

A BRIEF DIAGNOSIS OF THE INDIVIDUAL CASES

ALTHOUGH the cases of colour-blindness which were tested have been discussed in connection with the tests, the discussion has been hampered by the massing of results. It will be instructive, therefore, to collect the data for each colour-blind, and give a brief diagnosis of each individual case as revealed by the tests.

Subject A :

A is a typical colour-blind. From different tests it has been gathered that she has a neutral band in the blue-green region of the spectrum. From Stilling's Tables it would appear that she has a shortened spectrum at the red end, for she is unable to read Table 3. This was confirmed by her confusion of blue with pink. She does not, however, mistake red for black. The subject can distinguish highly saturated greens and reds, but has always experienced great difficulty with pale colours; yellows, fawns, pale pinks, and pale greens, are constantly confused. The subject has always been aware of her difficulty in this respect. In the wool test, we saw that the matches to the vivid green and the vivid red were excellent; it was only when the paler colours were reached that the confusion began to make its appearance. On being asked to divide out all the skeins into bundles, she placed together blues and violets; greens, yellows and fawns; greens, moles and greys; greens and browns ; light greens and yellows ; pale green and pink. She distinguished the reds, however, from the blue-reds.

All through the tests, it has been confirmed again and again that certain reds are visible to her. How otherwise can we explain the result that in the Nagel card test, in the Edridge-Green lantern, in the wool test, and in others, red can be distinguished ? In the colour naming, too, the bright red dots in Stilling's Tables are clearly recognized.

It would seem, however, that red is much better recognized than green, and that the blindness to green is the greater. The green when it inclines to a blue-green is seen as a grey, but otherwise there is a constant confusion with yellow. Apparently Dr Ladd-Franklin's description would just fit the case, namely, that " red vision had ' fallen out ' and green vision had been turned into yellow vision," were it possible for the red vision not to have " fallen out " entirely.

A, of course, does not always recognize red, for she sometimes calls it green, as we saw with the Edridge-Green lantern. And signal-green appeared to her almost white. In after-images the red stimulus gave a white after-image, but the green stimulus gave a red after-image. In coloured shadows the red shadow was correctly named, but the green shadow was mistaken for red, and the yellow one was called green. In the rings contrast, the red contrast colour was seen, but the green one only appeared grey. In the coloured diagram, the reds were correctly matched, but the greens were matched with greys, lavenders and blues, while greens were confused with browns. In the Bradley Paper Test it was always the greens and greys that showed confusion. In colour-mixing the blue-green was matched with a grey, and the green with a yellow, but the red had to be considerably diluted before it could be matched with a grey. These results cannot all be accidental, but the curious fact is, that if Stilling's Tables are correct then her sensibility to red should be weakened, as the red end of the spectrum is shortened. The only confirmation of this is the confusion of blue with pink. But the results taken as a whole would indicate that the shortening cannot be extensive, as we failed to find any other evidence of it.

Our final finding is that the subject is a red-green colour-blind. She is not entirely red-green colour-blind, for we do not find that she is entirely unable to see these colours. She makes the typical mistakes of the colour-blind, but under favourable circumstances, if the colour be of a certain hue, red and green can both be distinguished. The blindness to red, moreover, is less severe than the blindness to green, for the former colour is better identified.

Subject B :

This subject presents a somewhat similar case, and his chief difficulty lies with the pale colours. Since being tested, he has discovered that his brother suffers from a like defect, and makes the same kind of mistakes as the subject does.

B is a red-green colour-blind with normal length of spectrum, and a neutral band in the blue-green. He is an extremely careful subject, and matched the skeins in the wool test with great care and, to outward appearance, with great difficulty. He confuses greens, fawns and yellows, and pale greens with pale pinks. Very often in choosing skeins he lifts one up, lays it side by side with the test skein, and after long deliberation accepts or rejects it. He spontaneously gives his opinion of the confusion skein, saying whether lighter or darker. The magenta skein he matched with all shades of blue and violet, which clearly showed a deficiency in red. He can frequently detect differences in colours, such as violet and blue, or even magenta and crimson ; for it is impossible to get these equated on a colour-mixer. He is one of those who require the addition of a third disc of blue in equating red and green equal to grey. In matching blue-green with grey, his final equation does not give him entire satisfaction.

He seems to be more sensitive to red than A, for he recognizes the red in the coloured shadow, in the rings contrast, and in the after-images ; although he expresses doubt in the last case. In the Nagel card test, however, he includes card 11, with the reddish spots, showing a confusion of red with brown, and, further, he includes card 15—which only contains *two red spots*—in the reds only. He found this test one of great difficulty, but it is noteworthy that whenever a particular bright shade of red appeared, it was invariably identified.

The subject has greater difficulty with greens, and they are often confused with yellow. The shades of grey, however, in the Bradley papers, were all thought to be shades of green.

This subject yields a similar diagnosis to A's. He is a red-green colour-blind with, however, a normal length of spectrum and a small neutral band in the blue-green. He is not totally blind to red and green, for they can be seen if conditions are favourable.

Subject C :

This is a most curious case of colour-blindness, and it may be instructive to examine the results obtained from him with a little more detail than in the preceding cases.

In Stilling's Tables, the first Table reads :

| 56 | 27 | 89 | 43 |

the subject read :

| 86 | 28 | 89 | 48 |

Similarly in Table 2 we find :

| 39 | 42 | 86 | 75 |

the subject read :

| 88 | 48 | 88 | 75 |

These give evidence of colour weakness only, and at first the case was considered as showing, not blindness to colours, but a slight colour anomaly. The subject reads Table 3 correctly, but Tables 4, 5, 6, 7, 8, and 10 are beyond him.

In naming the colours of the spots on the Tables, it was found that a curious confusion existed in the subject's mind. Red and green were constantly mistaken, and the usual confusions of the colour-blind made their appearance. For example, in the first Table, which contains red figures on a green background, he described them as brown and dark green figures on a brown and a yellow background ; and if we trace his results all through the Tables we find the same confusion existing.

With Holmgren's wools he makes many mistakes, and finds the test a difficult one, for he is not at all sure of the colours of the skeins. Brown he matches with a very dark crimson and an emerald green, and throughout he makes the characteristic mistakes of the colour-blind. Here, again, his nomenclature is very faulty : test skein 1 he declares to be red, or yellow, or brown ; brown he calls very dark green ; pink he names green ; rose-pink he describes as green with red about it ; violets and purples he calls blue ; orange is thought to be yellow ; and he

P

often employs the term reddish-green. Red and green, too, are frequently confused.

Therefore it is all the more extraordinary to find that he can match colours with surprising accuracy on the colour wheel, and in the majority of cases he can obtain a normal equation. His naming of the colours while matching them shows much confusion, and yet his ultimate result is good. The equation, green and red and blue =grey, is almost identical with the normal equation. Attempts failed to match blue and violet, green and grey, red and grey, green and yellow ; in fact, no match could be obtained which would not be accepted by the normal eye. The matches in colour-mixings seem, therefore, to indicate perfect colour-vision, whereas atrocious nomenclature and mistakes in selecting wools seem to indicate red-green colour-blindness.

The other experiments emphasize the *defect*, and point to the subject being colour-blind. The Bradley Papers indicate weakness in the blue-green regions of the spectrum and a corresponding defect in the extra-spectral purples. The greys appear to him green. In the coloured shadows he sees both the red and green shadows as grey ; in the rings contrast, grey again is seen where red and green are clearly visible to the normal eye. The after-images likewise reveal a similar defect. The Nagel Card Test points to the defect being a grave one. No red dots at all are visible to him, and seven cards are said to contain green only, whereas but one of these is correct. The Edridge-Green Lantern confirms these results, and shows a hopeless confusion of colours. If the subject had been the correct distance away from the lantern, this result would have been greatly emphasized. In fact, the reduction of the aperture to No. 3 reduced most of the colours to a spot of light.

The evidence from these experiments, and the fact that he accepted the normal Rayleigh equation, place him among the colour-blinds.

Colour equations and Stilling's Tables are the only two tests which credit him with good colour-vision.   The other tests all point to the defect as one of red-green colour-blindness, with a normal length of spectrum, and a neutral band in the blue-greens.   It seems possible, therefore, for a colour-blind to avoid detection if Stilling's Tables are used alone.[1]

Subject D :

This subject is a "dangerous" colour-blind. He presents a somewhat similar case to that of C. He can partially pass Stilling's Tables, but his nomenclature shows considerable confusion.   Pale blue he calls brown or green ; pale pink, he sees as grey or yellow ; violet he calls blue ; and in selecting the wools, much confusion is exhibited, and the usual mistakes of the red-green colour-blind are made.   When tested with colour-mixing, however, his results show great improvement. With the complementary red and green, he requires the addition of a third colour before he is satisfied.   It is impossible to get equations from him such as were obtained from some of the other colour-blinds.   In the coloured shadows experiment, the green shadow is recognized, but the red shadow is seen as yellow.   In the rings contrast, the red and green are seen as grey, but in the after-images both the red and the green images can be distinguished.   In the Nagel Card Test, he can only pick out three cards containing red spots, out of a possible ten. He can see none containing red spots only ; and he makes mistakes in picking

---

[1] Edridge-Green, in discussing colour-blindness, states :   "Many colour-blinds match correctly, but name the principal colours wrongly."

out the green and grey cards. With the Edridge-Green
Lantern he mistakes the purple disc for green ; a dull
foggy red is invisible to him ; green combined with
neutral 5, which to the normal eye appears red, is seen as
a green.

He is certainly colour-defective, but his acceptance of
the normal Rayleigh equation prevents his inclusion in
the class of " anomalous trichromates." He must be
classed as a red-green colour-blind.   His Rayleigh equation
is : 200 red + 160 green = 38 yellow + 57 white + 265
black.   Compare this with his equation of red and green
= grey : 118·5 red + 204·5 green + 37 blue = 264 black
+ 96 white. The former shows an excess of red beyond
the normal ; the latter, an excess of green.

There is no doubt, however, that, under certain conditions, red and green may be visible to him (but they are
not always recognized as such).   He seems a mild case of
colour-blindness, milder even than A or B.

Subject E :

This subject from cumulative evidence appears to have
a large neutral band embracing the greens and the blue-
greens.   In the Stilling's test he is unable to read Tables
1 and 2, but reads Table 3, which suggests that he has a
spectrum of normal length.   From the spectral diagnosis
and the Bradley Papers, it seems probable, however, that
the spectrum is a little shortened at the red end, and it is
interesting to note that this conclusion is confirmed by
Professor Roaf's spectral diagnosis of his painting.

In matching the wools he does the vivid red and the
vivid green correctly, although in making the latter match
he was seen to examine and reject a pink.   The medium
greens and pinks show the typical colour-blind confusion
with one another and with yellows and browns.   The

medium pink appears almost a white to the subject, and to obtain suitable matches is a task of extreme difficulty. The magenta skein is matched with bluish pinks, blues and violets.

His nomenclature shows the typical confusion. For example, in the first of Stilling's Tables, he describes the red figures on the green background as violet on grey. The second Table, which .reverses the same colours, is described as green on grey. He shows a further confusion of red with brown, and green with fawn and mole. Naming the wools gives like results ; orange is mistaken for yellow, purple for blue, violet for pink, pink and green for grey. A colour is often described as a blue-grey, a green-grey, a red-grey ; and the term " flesh-colour " is often utilized.

The coloured shadows are rightly discriminated, although the yellow is described as brown. In the rings contrast the pink is not recognized ; the green and the yellow are named greenish-grey and brownish-grey respectively. No after-images could be obtained from a red or a green stimulus.

The Nagel Card Test he finds difficult, and he had to trace each ring round with a pencil before making a decision. In selecting cards with red spots, he chooses No. 12, which Nagel states is almost complete evidence of colour-blindness ; the brown spots on this card he mistakes for red. This same card is selected later as containing green spots only. Similar mistakes in selecting grey only and red only are made.

In the colour equations he can obtain a satisfactory match with red and green equalling grey without the addition of the blue disc. A similar equation can be obtained for blue and yellow. This latter equation—perfect to E—appears decidedly pink and green to the normal eye. He matched blue-green with grey, but not green with yellow. This can be explained if the neutral

band extends to the green.   Thus it is seen as grey, and
not as yellow.   The subject cannot get rid of the brown
tint in the yellow. Violet is matched with blue, but red
cannot be equated with green, nor with yellow and black.

In the Edridge-Green Lantern red often appears as
brown ; yellow is sometimes green, sometimes red, sometimes brown; violet is seen as blue.   Although signal-
green itself is seen as green, yet when modified by neutral
4 or neutral 5, it appears as grey.   Pure green + N.5 is
seen as grey-brown, and pure green alone appears a light
brown.   Yellow alone may be called a light brown ; but
a double disc of yellow changes the colour to red.   Aperture
3 changes the colours red A, red B, yellow, pure green,
signal-green, blue, violet, to red, orange, brown, green,
dark grey, red-blue, red.

Yellow and blue are clearly recognized ; red and green
seem sometimes to be recognized.   It is interesting in
this subject's case to note, however, that pale blue is at
times seen as a grey, and that violet is more than once
described as a dark grey.   There is a possibility of a
shortening of the spectrum at the violet end, probably
similar to the shortening at the red end.

Subject F :

This subject cannot read the first 12 Tables in Stilling's
Tests, although he occasionally reads a figure here and
there.   This would suggest he was blue-yellow blind as
well as red-green blind, which he certainly is not.   He
appears to be red-green blind with slight shortening of
the spectrum at the red end, and there is a suggestion of
a weakened sensitivity in the green as well as the
blue-green regions.

With the Holmgren wools, he shows confusion from the
beginning.   The vivid green he matches with greens,

yellows and drabs ; the vivid red with a vivid red skein, and a very dark green. The brown proved difficult to match ; with the magenta he put pinks, violets, blues, greens and greys. The medium and pale skeins showed the usual confusion. With the pale blue he invariably matched blues and pinks—and this confusion extended to the darker shades of red as well.

In colour-naming he makes many mistakes. Red is confused with fawn and mole, drab and brown, and very often with blue. Green is often taken for yellow or pink. What is very characteristic of this subject, however, is his vague, indefinite phraseology in describing colours, which we noted in the colour-naming tests. " Some red in it," " red and something else," etc. A grey skein of wool he describes as " red and something else, perhaps brown."

The Nagel Card Test he finds difficult and he shows great confusion of green with red both in selecting the proper cards in Section A and in naming the cards in Section B. In the coloured shadow test, the red shadow is seen correctly, but the green is described as red. A similar result appears in the rings contrast. The after-image of yellow is described as blue or red, that of red as white, and that of green as blue.

In colour-mixing he requires the third disc of blue in matching the complementary colours, red and green, but his final equation shows a marked deviation from the normal. He matches red and blue-green with grey, green with yellow, orange with yellow, and violet with blue.

The Edridge-Green Lantern was a severe test for him, and he took longer to test than any of the other subjects. He finds the red especially trying. Red A is thought to be yellow, and red B a yellowish brown. Very often signal-green is confused with red, and when combined with neutral 5, it becomes invisible. Pure green is seen as yellow, but neutral 5 placed before it changes it to red. Neutral 4 and neutral 5, both reddish, are seen as green by the subject. Purple and N.4, which give a full red, he can hardly see. The reduction of the aperture to 3 causes the colours to appear as spots of light, except those of blue and violet, which he recognizes as blues.

This case shows a greater defect than that of A or B. It was discovered by chance in the playing of a game in which colours had to be distinguished ; but the subject was quite unaware of any abnormality in his colour-vision.

Subject G :

G was unaware of his defect until tested, and accordingly was loath to admit its presence. He is a difficult subject to test, for he tries as much as possible to cover his failings. His spectrum is of normal length (there may be a slight shortening at the red end), with a neutral band extending over the green and blue-green.

He fails completely to read Tables 1 and 2 of Stilling's Test, but reads 3 without difficulty. In naming the colour of the dots and the wools, he makes the typical mistakes of a red-green colour-blind. In matching the test skeins of wools he selects his colours with great deliberation, but, notwithstanding all his caution, he betrays his defect by making the characteristic confusions. With the vivid red, he places pinks, drabs, greys and blues. He can give no match to the pale pink skein, for it appears to him as a " dirty white." The medium green and pink are matched with a large variety of wools of different hues.

The following colour-mixings are successful : green with grey, red with grey, violet with blue. Red is matched with green, both discs diluted, but the two colours clearly visible to a normal eye. No third disc is required in equating red and green with grey, nor blue and yellow with grey. Green cannot be matched with yellow, which may be explained by the presence of a neutral band there.

In the Nagel Card Test, he is able to find only two cards containing reddish spots, can find none with red or grey only, but selects 14 cards containing green alone, only one of which is correct. In Section B of the same test he commits many errors.

In the coloured shadows red and green are invisible, but the yellow appears green. The green in the rings contrast is seen as dark grey, the red as blue. Red and green stimuli only result in grey after-images.

The Edridge-Green Lantern reveals his defect very prettily, for the modifying glasses are troublesome to him. Red A and red B can be distinguished, but, with a neutral glass in front, they become green every time. The first four neutral glasses are seen as reds, but neutral 5 is a green. If in doubt as to a colour, green is the name preferred. Yellow is a difficult colour for him, and is usually confused with red, particularly when a red precedes it. The ground glass is especially trying for G, and it is noticeable that when such a modifying glass is used, he spends a very long time coming to a decision. It seems to change the colour completely, and causes an erroneous answer to be made.

G seems to be able sometimes to distinguish red and green, but neither is a clear sensation for him, and they are both liable to be confused with one another or with some other colour.

Subject H :

This subject is a limiting case of dichromasy : his only sensations are those of blue and yellow. Red and green are totally invisible, and under no circumstances can they be recognized. His spectrum shows a shortening at the red end, with a neutral band embracing the green and the blue-green. From cumulative evidence, the violet end of the spectrum appears to be cut off to a small extent. From the colour-mixings it is seen that red, orange, yellow and grass green appear as nuances of yellow, blue and violet as nuances of blue. His nomenclature is very constant—red is called black, but, if a little diluted, is termed a brown. Green is seen as grey, but a bright green with a touch of yellow in it is termed orange.

It is noteworthy that in the Nagel Card Test, he fails completely in Section A ; no red spots at all can be found, for they all appear to him as blue. No card containing green spots only can be selected, and the card with nothing but red spots is picked out as of a uniform grey.

Red is not seen once when he is tested with the lantern, and signal-green appears white. The modifying glass causes no change in colour, but suggests a difference in shade. Grey is a frequent answer given, and orange, too, is employed on many occasions.

The coloured shadows reveal a total lack of red and green sensations, which result is confirmed in the rings contrast test and in the after-images. In all three tests red and green are replaced by grey.

With the Bradley Paper Test, a definite defect in shade is noticeable. This seems to be characteristic of a shortened spectrum.

This subject has two brothers who have monochromatic vision.

Subject I :

This subject is noteworthy for his remarkable nomenclature, and for the variety of colours which he confuses.

In the Stilling's Tables, 1 and 2 can be deciphered, but with extreme difficulty. Table 3 cannot be read at all. This indicates a shortened spectrum. The colours of this Table which are crimson on black and mole, are seen as dark grey on shades of grey. Crimson and red, as is to be expected, are frequently mistaken for black or dark grey.

In naming the wools, reddish-green is a term made use of on numerous occasions. He is seldom content with a single-colour name, but uses such phrases as " golden brown," and " crimson lake," the former applied to brownish or emerald greens, the latter to dark green. These terms are used with evident satisfaction. A threefold description is not unusual, and grey or dark violet may be termed as " pinkish-greenish-brownish." In matching the Holmgren wools he thought the brown skein was the vivid red one given to him again in mistake. The confusions he makes with the wools are numerous, and begin in the highly-saturated skeins. Vivid green is matched with greens, pinks, and browns ; vivid red with green, browns and blues. The other skeins reveal a like confusion.

It is difficult to get colours equated on the colour wheel, for his nomenclature is so misleading. In equating red and green with grey, a third disc is required, but the final equation contains only 68° red, as compared with the normal 113°, and contains a correspondingly large sector of green. Green and red diluted are both matched with grey, 197° of green compared with 195° of red, so that it is possible to match green directly with red. His equations are very similar to those of H, except that red cannot be equated with yellow and black. Green is matched with yellow and orange, and violet with blue.

It seems evident that this case is a red-green colour-blind, with shortened spectrum at the red end and probably at the violet end (for results tend to point to that conclusion), and a neutral band in the blue-greens. His colour sensations seem to be that of yellow and blue.

Subject J :

It will have been gathered from the tests that this subject is completely blind to red and green. In the centre he has a large neutral band embracing the yellow-greens, greens and blue-greens. The two colour sensations which he does experience seem to fill only a small part of the spectrum, and from the results of different tests it appears that there is a reduced sensitivity to these two colours. In the coloured shadows, the yellow cannot be discriminated, and the shadow, which appears vivid to the experimenter, is merely called grey. In other words, the yellow must be highly saturated before it is distinguished. A disc of yellow was rotated on a colour wheel and when diluted with a little white it was matched with a grey by the subject. $258°$ yellow $+ 102°$ white $= 92°$ black $+ 268°$ white. The yellow was distinctly visible in the final equation, but seemed to make no impression on the subject.

The large number of colour skeins, all selected as of the same hue, is remarkable ; and each time a skein is given, most of the wools are matched with it. In naming the dots in Stilling's Tables, he can perceive no colour, but monotonously maintains they are all " shades of grey." In naming the wools, too, the same result is apparent. We have already described his colour equations under experiment No. 4, giving examples of his colour matches. In the Lantern test, his answers were unfailingly " grey," and it was a relief sometimes to hear the name " blue," or even " black." Out of the 76 combinations shown, 50 of these were described as grey, 6 as black, 2 as white, while on six occasions nothing was experienced, giving a grand total of 64 colourless sensations.

In the Nagel Card Test, all sixteen cards in Section A are seen as grey, while the cards in Section B merely represent different shades of grey and black.

In the Bradley Paper Test, a grave defect in shade is apparent, evidently typical of a shortened spectrum. The red end of the spectrum is considerably shortened, and there seems to be an accompanying shortening of the violet end as well. This might be described as a case of colour-blindness, just preceding total, in which the yellow and blue regions have become restricted to narrow patches in the spectrum.

The subject's maternal grandmother had great difficulty with colours, and his uncle on the same side can distinguish highly saturated colours only, having great difficulty with pale colours. I tested his sister's vision, and found it to be perfectly normal. The subject discovered his defect while in the army, when he failed to distinguish S.O.S. signals while out on patrol.

An Anomalous Trichromate:

An anomalous trichromate was tested with Stilling's Tables. She was found able to read most of them, but made a few mistakes with No. 6 and No. 10. Her colour naming was excellent, both in the Tables and with the wools, nor did she make any confusions in selecting suitable matches. From the Rayleigh equation she was found

to be red anomalous, which was again verified in matches
of red and green with grey.

Rayleigh Equation : 208° red + 152° green =
Compare with 208 red + 99 green + 53 blue =

It is an interesting coincidence that the sections of red in
both equations are identical.

In the coloured shadows both red and green were
identified, but in the rings contrast the green was called
grey and the red purple.

There exists a hiatus between this case and the colour-
blinds, but it seems probable that the gap could be filled
by gradation cases with the defect step by step becoming
more serious and the confusion increasing. The case
appears the beginning of a defect in red, which one can
imagine increasing in severity until a milder form of colour-
blindness takes its place.

A second subject was tested—since the above was
written—who seems also well classed among the anomalous
trichromates. Her sensations of colour are considerably
weakened, and it is worthy of note that her father and
brothers suffer from colour-blindness.

The defect of this subject first came to light in an
experiment involving colour-mixing. The difficulties in
obtaining a match were very noticeable, and a long time
was spent in the adjustment of the discs. Finally, the
match given as perfect was not valid for the normal eye.
A further investigation with Stilling's Tables revealed—
not colour-blindness, but colour-weakness. The test
with Holmgren's wools did not indicate any serious
defect—although many omissions of skeins occurred—
nor did the test with the Bradley Papers reveal much
colour-anomaly. In the latter test, however, one fact
attracted considerable attention. It was obvious that

almost immediately on seeing the colours the eyes of the subject became extremely fatigued. The colours seemed to have a dazzling effect, and a rest pause had to be instituted after every choice of colour made. This fatigue was very marked, and the subject confessed that, after the colour-mixing experiment in class the previous week, her eyes had been very painful.

In the colour-mixing experiments tried as part of the investigation, the results of which are comparable with those of the colour-blinds tested, the following equations were obtained :—

$$127° \text{ green} + 233° \text{ white} = 56° \text{ black} + 304° \text{ white.}$$
$$138° \text{ red} + 222° \text{ white} = 83° \text{ black} + 277° \text{ white.}$$
$$360° \text{ violet} = 135° \text{ blue} + 225° \text{ black.}$$

From these results it is evident that there is a slight weakness to both green and red, for in the first two equations, where both these colours are matched with greys, they were not—to the normal eye—totally eliminated by the admixture of white, but, though pale, were clearly visible. The matching of violet with blue was rather a surprise to the experimenter, who had not judged the colour defect serious enough to give this particular colour equation.

With the Edridge-Green Lantern test, one or two mistakes were made. It is worthy of note that this test apparently caused little or no fatigue. The yellow disc (which approximates to orange) was difficult to describe, and at last was recognized as a " pure colour between grey and white." This disc was always identified when it appeared, but no more definite name could be assigned to it ; when two yellows were shown, however, the name given was yellowish brown. Neutral 1, which diminishes the intensity of light, could not be distinguished. What *was* described as yellow was neutral 4, which resembles red more than yellow.

Greens, when modified by neutral glasses, caused difficulty, and were often thought to be greys. Signal-green itself was confused with blue. Violet also, was invariably mistaken for blue, although the purple disc was more or less correctly described. Red was sometimes mistaken for yellow. Weakened sensitivity to red, green, and perhaps yellow, seems to be the conclusion to be drawn from this test.

This case accordingly differs from the anomalous tri-chromate described above. It seems to be slightly more severe, and the green is affected as well as the red. It seems possible to imagine the defect in this case growing more pronounced, with the red and green gradually losing in sensitivity until partial colour-blindness is revealed. This case forms, it may be, a further link between an anomalous trichromate and a colour-blind. So small is the defect relatively that the subject was unaware of its existence until tested, but, in the cursory examination given, the defect was clearly substantiated by the results obtained from the colour equations and the Edridge-Green Lantern.

From the analysis of the colour-blinds, one fact stands clearly out, that the sensations which they experience most distinctly are blue and yellow. Certainly, in the case of the last three subjects, these are the only colours visible to them. Dr Pole, in describing his own case of colour-vision, made this quite clear, and the diagnosis of his spectrum might well be that of H.[1] " The most salient fact in dichromic vision is its remarkably simple and symmetrical character, consisting of one pair of comple-mentary colours, with gradations of nuance perfectly

[1] *Transactions of the Royal Society of Edinburgh*, Vol. 37.

symmetrically disposed." Appended below (Figure VIII) is the circular diagram for normal vision, drawn first by

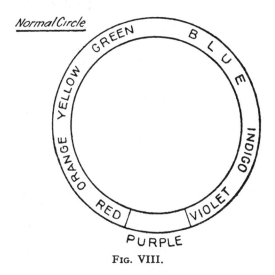

FIG. VIII.

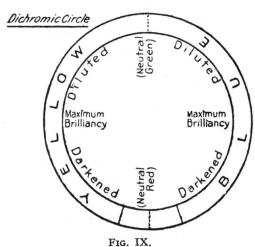

FIG. IX.

Newton and perfected by Donders in 1881. Figure IX was constructed on similar principle, to represent the dichromic spectrum, and Pole describes it thus: " In

Q

this the pair of visible colours are shown with their maxima diametrically opposite, and from these two points they become modified, in one direction by darkening only, in the other by darkening combined with dilution, till, at the top and bottom, the colours meet, and become lost in the neutral points. And these two neutral points, also diametrically opposite each other, correspond to the other pair of complementary colours, the purple-red and blue-green, which, though most prominent colours to the normal-eyed, are invisible colours to the colour-blind. It will be at once seen what a remarkable symmetry this structure presents, and how greatly the regular arrangement of the dichromic series of colour impressions differs from the irregular structure of the normal series in the adjacent figure."

This diagram has been accepted by more than one investigator as being true to fact. It certainly only meets such extreme cases as those of subject H, in which the spectrum left of the neutral band appears yellow, and right of the neutral band is seen as blue. Yet even in his case the neutral band would require to be extended over the green as well as the blue-green. J, however, would require a modified diagram, for red and green with him are not replaced by yellows, but by grey. (See Figure X.) His sensations of colour have one point of resemblance with those of H, in that they are similar in hue. The one difference is that they vary in extent, and only cover a very small portion of the spectrum. This distinctly shows the large variety which exists among colour-blinds. These two may be regarded as extreme cases, and yet they present entirely different features, for the one has a much larger colour range, if we may so term it, than the other. It, therefore, seems unprofitable to systematize the colour sensations of the colour-blind, so many individual types exist.

Moreover, a totally different diagram would be required for the milder cases of dichromasy, for not only are yellow and blue visible to them, but red and green, too, if circumstances are favourable. They agree with the diagram, however, in so far that yellow and blue are distinct sensations to them, which are never confused with one another,

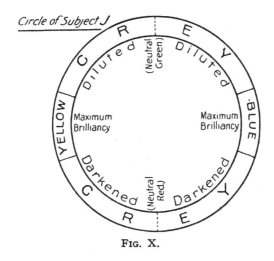

FIG. X.

no matter how grave or how mild the defect ; but the diagram gives a false impression of cases where these two sensations are not the only ones existent. Allowance must be made for these less extreme cases, which we have been describing, and which appear to be more prevalent than the limiting types.

CHAPTER VII

1. *Colours Confused by the Colour-Blind*

1. Confusion of red with black : This indicates shortening of the red end of the spectrum.

2. Confusion of violet with black: This indicates shortening of the violet end.[1] If the violet is not always so confused, or is only confused when the colour is at a distance, the shortening is not very great. (This fact emerges in the cases E, H, I, and J.)

3. Confusion of blue with black : This occurred only once with subject I. It may be accidental, for it is rarely met with ; it would suggest a neutral band in the blue.

4. Confusion of a colour with grey : This indicates a neutral band in that respective colour. Blue-green we found was often mistaken for grey ; likewise red.

5. Confusion of blue with pink : This, as has already been pointed out, indicates a shortened spectrum.

6. Other common confusions, all characteristic of the defect, are :   red with green
green with brown
red with brown
green with yellow
most pale colours with one another.

7. Green may be confused with purple, owing to a second neutral band beyond the spectrum.

---

[1] The shortening of the violet end of the spectrum may have a different explanation. It may be caused by the second neutral band extending as far as and into the violet.

8. Red may be invisible to the individual, or may be replaced by yellow ; likewise green.

2. *Constancy of Colours for the Colour-Blind*

The colour-blind do not guess colours as is very generally supposed. They have a definite system of colour sensations which often prevents their detection. It has been made generally clear from the results discussed, that the examinees were regulating their answers by their own experiences. The case of H and his use of the term " orange " provides an excellent example.

One other fact stands out clearly in this connection. With some subjects a colour name is appropriated and is used with such frequency as to become almost an idiosyncrasy. E's particular phrase is " yellowish-brown," F's is " flesh-colour," I's use of " crimson lake " and " golden brown " may also be submitted as striking examples.

3. *Some Characteristics of the Colour-Blind*

1. They are more sensitive to contrast effects than the normal. This was clearly indicated in the Lantern test.

2. They show quicker fatigue to colours than the normal. The case of J is the strongest example, for fatigue was noticeably present when he was tested with the Bradley Papers. B, too, in the after-image test, had to rest his eyes for quite a long period before a fresh stimulus could be presented.

3. In cases of shortened spectrum, there may exist a defective shade perception, due to the absence of the red rays.

4. Some colour-blinds try to conceal their defect and employ every device they can think of to this end.

5. A modification in intensity of light is for the colour-blind a change of colour.

4. Bearing of Results on Theories of Colour-Vision

It is not proposed in this section to assert dogmatically that the results fit in with any particular theory. It was explained in the Introduction that the experiments were carried out without any preconceived theory causing a bias, and the question now arises, how far do the results tell for or against existing theories?

Although we have considerable admiration for Dr Edridge-Green's practical achievements, which have been productive of much valuable information and many useful tests, it must be admitted that his theory of colour-vision is difficult to reconcile with facts. It has been found impossible to group the ten subjects into specific unit classes. H and J may be grouped as two-units, although we should be very loath to admit that red and violet are the two colours visible to them. It somewhat disarms criticism to find that, according to Edridge-Green, they are not supposed to see these two colours, but only the centres of their two psycho-physical units which are yellow and blue. Even admitting this, subject J raises a difficulty. He appears an extreme case of red-green colour-blindness with his yellow and blue sensations reduced in sensitivity. In fact, he may be regarded as akin to, or as just preceding monochromatic vision. If so, and if Edridge-Green's theory is understood correctly, should not red and violet, the two extremes of the spectrum, be the colours visible to J? Further, if the centre colours of the units are always the colours seen, then the colour sensations of the colour-blind must vary from individual to individual, since the position of their psycho-physical units varies. In fact, a shortening of the spectrum at either end will narrow the band of colour and shift the centre. J has shortened spectrum at the red end, a large neutral band, a small region of yellow, a second neutral band, a small region of blue, and the violet end shortened. There is no suggestion whatsoever that red and violet are the colours he sees, and certainly yellow does not form the centre of his red, nor blue the centre of his violet. It seems quite clear that yellow and blue are the two colours seen, and that these colours are the last seen before monochromatic vision supervenes.

When we come to the three-units, the same difficulty arises. We find that reddish-green is a term used by the three-unit; therefore, we try to place B in the three-unit class, from that and other evidence, but without success. The three colours of the three-unit class are red, green, and violet. The three-unit never confuses red with green, but is always in difficulty with yellows and blues. This seems contrary to fact. B, or any of the other subjects examined, is always confusing red with green, but yellow and blue are two of his clearest sensations. The confusion of brown with green is a diagnostic sign of the four-unit. This class can see clearly red, yellow, green, and violet, but here again the facts point to different conclusions. The results, therefore, as we have found them, are difficult to reconcile with this theory, and rather appear to give direct evidence against it.

As a further point of explanation, it may be argued that yellow and blue are not clearly seen by the three-unit, that yellow is frequently confused with green, and blue with violet, as Edridge-Green affirms. This is true, but it appears to be a begging of the question. Yellow is confused with green in cases where the green element is absent, as in a compound of yellow-green, or in cases of colour-blindness where green has been replaced by yellow and called green by convention, but that does not alter the statement that yellow is a distinct colour sensation.

Blue, likewise, shows confusion with violet and with pink, but is not that because the red element is not recognized in these two cases. It does not affect the validity of the statement that blue is a clear colour sensation of the red-green colour-blind.

In the Ladd-Franklin theory, the red element "falls out" in red-blindness, and green is replaced by yellow; in green-blindness the green element "falls out" and yellow replaces red.

In the results submitted, certain cases seem partially to support this theory; whether they wholly support it is difficult to decide. One fact, which does give it support in the extreme cases, is that yellow and blue are the only two colours visible. In H and J's cases the red and green must both have fallen out and been replaced by yellow; in other words, there has been a total regression to the second stage.

It seems more difficult to account for the milder forms. With some of the examinees green is replaced by yellow, which would appear to support the theory; this occurs in cases of red-blindness or in those cases in which the spectrum is shortened. But we have repeatedly shown that red is not totally invisible, nor green either. Therefore, all the red cannot have "fallen out," nor all the green been replaced by yellow.

In green-blindness, the green sensation is said to be missing, and yellow vision takes the place of the red. The same argument holds here, for the red is not always replaced by yellow, nor does the green element always appear to be missing. In fact, the division of colour-blinds into two such groups seems unnatural and essentially artificial.[1] There is little difference between a case of

[1] Dr Houston's results, of which the writer has just become aware, confirm this statement (*vide* p. 224).

shortened spectrum and a case in which the spectrum is of normal length when milder forms of the defect are in question. For in our results there seems little difference between A and B, although the former is credited with a shortening of the spectrum. It may be that Dr Ladd-Franklin has modified her theory to explain such cases, but so far attempts to find a reference to such modification have failed.

The " old " explanation of Helmholtz may be set aside, for the newer explanation fits the facts much better. It must be admitted that few text-books on the subject seem to recognize or acknowledge this second mode of explanation, and still give Helmholtz's views along the line which he himself so vigorously repudiated.

In red-blindness—that is, in cases of shortened spectrum —the red substance has become equal to the green substance ; but yellow and blue are the two colours visible. The yellow begins in the orange, and the blue-green forms the neutral band. In green-blindness, the opposite condition occurs, and the neutral band appears in the green.

This theory, while accounting for some of the facts, seems again to make an unnatural division between colour-blinds and not to make any allowance for the type of case we have been describing, or those described by Professor Hayes. Even McDougall's modification seems to fail to account for these red-green colour-blind cases in which these two colours may sometimes be recognized. If colour-blindness is atavistic, and facts seem to confirm that hypothesis, these cases may be regarded as midway between normal vision and total reversion to the blue-yellow stage. The great point of superiority of Edridge-Green's theory is that he recognizes such transitional cases.

Helmholtz's theory admirably fits the facts for extreme cases, those cases in which blue and yellow are the colour sensations experienced. It also gives a satisfactory reason why the neutral band should lie in the blue-green in red-blindness and in the green in green-blindness. Yet subjects H and J, as far as we were able to discover, appeared to have a neutral band embracing both. They are neither red-blind nor green-blind, but are red-green blind. It does not seem, however, to explain the milder cases of partial colour-blindness, unless it may be possible to account for them along the lines of Peddie by the formation of some derived colour triangle which will conform to the facts.

The Hering theory exposes itself to the same objection, namely, that it explains solely the limiting cases. It has the apparent advantage that red-green blindness is treated as a whole and is not so artificially divided into the types of Helmholtz. The variations, which do undoubtedly exist in this defect, are accounted for by differences in the pigmentation of the eye, and Hering decided, on the basis of experimental results, that colour-blinds could be regarded as yellow-sighted or blue-sighted. We have little evidence in favour of, or against, this view.

One outstanding result which does support the Hering theory is that the position of the neutral bands of the colour-blinds corresponds with the fundamental colours adopted in the theory. The one neutral band lies in the blue-green which is the green of the Hering theory ; the other lies in the complementary of that green, in the purples, which is the red employed by Hering—a red beyond the red end of the spectrum. These facts lend strong support to the theory in the fundamental colours chosen, for if the substances for these two elementary colours are absent, then the colour sense must be deficient in red and green, leaving as clear sensations the other two fundamental colours, blue and yellow.

Finally, our tentative finding is that the Hering theory, the Young-Helmholtz theory, and the Ladd-Franklin theory all fit the facts of red-green colour-blindness when the defect takes an extreme form, but they seem to fail to take account of cases which suffer from this disability in a less marked degree.

5. *Percentage of Colour-Blinds*

Five schools were examined in different districts of Edinburgh, involving the testing of over 1,000 children, whose ages ranged from 9 years to 12 years inclusive. The children were examined in groups by means of Stilling's Tables. They were supplied with pencils and paper, and were asked to write down the figures they saw.

Age.	*Colour-Blindness.*	
	Girls.	*Boys.*
9	0	1
10	1	4
11	2	4
12	1	2

Above gives a total of 4 girls out of 575 or ·6%, and 11 boys out of 563, or 1·9%. Four schools were mixed, and the fifth was a boys' school ; it yielded the largest number of cases, about one in each class of 30 pupils or slightly over 3%. The school which showed the next largest proportion was a mixed school in one of the poorest parts of the city, and it was this school which curiously enough yielded more girls' cases than boys', 3 girls out of the 88 tested.

When it is recalled that the complete total for girls for all the schools is only 4, the result is more amazing, but probably it is merely accidental. The other schools showed no connection between the defect and social status.

It is important that tests for colour-blindness should be inaugurated in the schools, so that the children's parents may become acquainted with the defect. The detection of colour is involved in so many occupations that it is a waste of time and opportunity training a boy or girl for some particular vocation which may afterwards be found to be unsuitable. The literature of the subject abounds with instances of difficulties and hardships which apprentices have undergone because of their failure to see certain necessary colours. To quote a few instances of occupations unsuitable for those suffering from this disability will make this quite apparent : physician, chemist, artist, weaver, upholsterer, tailor, milliner, florist, the navy, the railway, the post-office, and so on. This constitutes quite a formidable and startling list, and although the discrimination of colours may not be absolutely essential in some of these vocations, the lack of it may lead to serious error.

In school, too, it must cause great inconvenience to the child. One of the subjects related how he remembered being dismissed from a drawing class at school by an irate master who thought he was amusing himself when mixing colours. The defect was not realized until the subject attended the secondary school, where his defect was discovered by the mathematical master in a curious manner. In geometry coloured chalks were used to differentiate between two triangles on the blackboard. The master naturally spoke of the red triangle and the green triangle, but the subject became greatly confused, and found it impossible to follow the explanation. To remedy matters, the subject was brought nearer, as the cause was attributed to bad eyesight, with, however, no better result. Some time later it occurred to the master that there existed some defect in colour, which was causing the difficulty, and the mystery was solved.

This is a single isolated instance, but instances could be multiplied indefinitely. It is essential that teachers should be aware that such a disability exists and the form it assumes. The testing of children in schools cannot be too strongly recommended. The Stilling's Tables make a very suitable group test by means of which " abnormals " can be detected and then examined more thoroughly to confirm the previous finding and diagnose the extent of the anomaly.

It may be advisable to give an account of the percentage of colour-blind from some authenticated source, for comparison, and for practical purposes. The percentage given by different investigators has varied slightly, but one fact stands out clearly—the frequency with which this defect occurs in men, and the limited number of cases which have been reported among women.

In an article by Thomson and Weiland[1] is given the interesting Table on page 223 which shows the prevalence of the defect among males of different nationalities, and the few cases which have been reported among women.

The percentage of colour-blinds in the male population is about 3·5, while in the female population it is only 0·088. This list can be supplemented from Jeffries,[2] who devotes an entire chapter to this question, quoting

[1] Norris and Oliver, *System of Diseases of the Eye.*
[2] *Colour-Blindness: its Dangers and its Detection.*

	Males Examined	Colour Blind	per cent.	Females Examined	Colour Blind	per cent.
Holmgren	32,165	1,019	3·16			
Jeffries	19,183	802	4·12	14,764	11	0·073
Committee of the Ophthalmological Society of Eng- land	14,846	617	4·16	489	2	0·4
Fontenay in Den- mark	4,000	155	3·8			
Dr Adele Field in China	600	19	3·16	600	1	0·17
In two Japanese regiments	1,200	41	3·4			
Total ...	71,994	2,653	3·69	15,853	14	0·088

result after result of percentages from extensive examina-
tions carried out by different investigators. Edridge-
Green objects to these results because they are mainly
based on examination with the Holmgren wool test. His
results, however, tally with the above percentage, for he
also gives the percentage of colour-blinds as 3·5, which
he considers near enough for practical purposes. Some
mention may be made here of the way in which colour-
blindness is inherited. Usually it is transmitted from
grandfather to grandson, whilst the mother of the son
remains free from the defect. Dr Pliny Earle in 1845[1]
reported the colour-blindness of four generations of his
own family. In the fourth generation, from 17 marriages,
there were 32 male descendants, 18 of whom were colour-
blind. Of the 29 females, only 2 were colour-blind. In
the third generation no colour anomaly is reported, showing
how colour-blindness may pass over one generation but
reappear in the succeeding one. In the cases of the two
colour-blinds in the fifth generation neither parents nor

[1] *American Journal of the American Sciences.*

grandparents showed the defect, showing here an interval of two generations.

Horner's Law (based on the tracing of cases of transmission of the defect by Professor Horner, of Zürich) seems to have been generally substantiated—at least his observations have been verified by different observers. His general conclusions are :—

(a) That colour-blind fathers have normal-eyed sons.

(b) That colour-blind sons have normal-eyed fathers.

(c) That sons of daughters whose father was colour-blind are most likely to be the same, although not without exception : or colour-blindness is transmitted from grandfather to grandchild.

The hereditary nature of colour-blindness is unquestioned ; usually each colour-blind can tell of a brother or some other relative who suffers from a similar defect to his own.

Dr Houston's Investigations

The results of Dr R. A. Houston, of Glasgow University, have just been brought to our notice.[1] He has adopted a new method of testing colour-blinds described by him as a " microscope " test. His conclusion is that he finds it impossible to separate his subjects into two classes or even to recognize two pronounced types such as advocated by Helmholtz. " The fundamental characteristic of the system of Helmholtz and Maxwell was that the colour sensations of the normal could be represented on a plane, whereas the sensations of the colour-blind required only a line or a point. All my cases require plane diagrams. Thus it follows that the colour-blind are trichromatics."

[1] *Proceedings of the Royal Society of Edinburgh*, Vol. 42, 1922.

We are not prepared to accept this without qualification, for our subjects H and J cannot possibly be trichromatic. It has been proved throughout all the experiments that they are true dichromates. But the statement supports the diagnoses of our other cases, in which we have repeatedly asserted that their colour sensations are not restricted to blue and yellow, but that sometimes green, at other times red, becomes visible to them. This finding of Dr Houston supports Professor Hayes' results, and incidentally our own conclusions.

BIBLIOGRAPHY

LIST OF WORKS, EDITIONS, AND PASSAGES TO WHICH
REFERENCE, OR OF WHICH USE HAS BEEN MADE

Abney, W. de W., " Colour-Blindness and the Trichromatic
Theory of Colour-Vision," *Proc. of Royal Soc.*, Dec.,
1910.
—— " On the Examination for Colour of Cases of
Tobacco Scotoma and of Abnormal Colour-Blindness,"
Proc. of Royal Soc., 49, 1891, 491–508.
—— *Colour-Vision*, London, 1895.
—— *Phil. Trans. Royal Soc.*, 1899, 100–3, 259; 1905, 105,
333.
—— *Researches in Colour-Vision and the Trichromatic
Theory*, London, 1913.
Abney and Festing, " Colour Photometry," 3, *Phil. Trans.*,
1892, 183, A, 531–65.
Aitken, J., *Proc. Roy. Scottish Soc. Arts*, 1871–72.
Allen, Frank, " Persistence of Vision in Colour-Blind Sub-
jects," *Phys. Rev.*, 15, 1905, 193–225.
Allen, Grant, *The Colour Sense*, London, 1892.
Ayers, E., " Colour-Blindness with Special Reference to
Art and Artists," *Cent. Mag.*, 73, 1907, 876–89.
Baird, J. W., *Colour Sensitivity of the Peripheral Retina*,
Carnegie Institute, Wash., 1905.
—— " The Problems of Colour-Blindness," *Psych. Bull.*,
5, 1908, 294–300.
Barret, G. W., " Problem of the Visual Requirements of
the Sailor and the Railway Employee," *Report Brit.
for the Adv. of Science*, 1914, 256–63.
Bell, L., " Types of Abnormal Colour-Vision," *Proc. Amer.
Acad.*, 1914, 1–13.
Bowditch, H., " Red-Green Colour-Blindness in Three Allied
Families," *Journ. of Heredity*, 13, 3, 139–42.
Bronner, E., " Colour-Blindness," *Med. Times and Gazette*,
1856.
Burch, G. F., *Memorandum Prepared for the Committee.
Minutes of Evidence*, 1912, 142–7.

227

Burch, G. F., " A Confusion Test for Colour-Blindness,"
Proc. Royal Soc., 1912, 81–3.

Burton-Opitz, R., *A Text-book of Physiology*, Philadelphia,
1920.

Butler, T. H., " On the Futility of the Official Tests for
Colour-Blindness," *Brit. Med. Journ.*, 1910, 316–7.

Calkins, M., *Introduction to Psychology*, London, 1901.

Chevreul, M. E., *On Colour*, London, 1859.

Clerk Maxwell, J., *Scientific Papers*, Cambridge, 1890.

—— " Experiments on Colour Perceived by the Eye, with
Remarks on Colour-Blindness," *Trans. Royal Soc.
Edin.*, 21, 1855, 275–297. (*See* Maxwell.)

Collins, G. L., *Colour-Blindness ; its Relation to Other Ocular
Conditions, and the Bearing on Public Health of Tests
of Colour Sense Acuity*, Pub. Health Bull. No. 92,
Wash. Gov. Print. Office, 1918.

Combe, G., *A System of Phrenology*, 1st Ed., 1830.

le Conte, *Sight*, Int. Scientific Series, London, 1895.

Dalton, J., " Extraordinary Facts Relating to the Vision of
Colours," *Trans. Lit. and Phil. Soc.*, Manchester, 1794.

Delabarre, E. B., " Coloured Shadows," *Amer. Journ. of
Psych.*, 2, 1888–9, 636–43.

Donders, F. C., *Annales d'Oculistique*, 34, 1880, 212.

Edridge-Green, F. W., *Trans. Ophth. Soc.*, 22, 1902.

—— Art., " Colour-Vision and Colour-Blindness," *Encyc.
Brit.*, 12th Ed., Vol. XXX.

—— *Journ. of Physiology*, 41, 1910.

—— *Proc. Royal Soc.*, B82, 1910, 456 ; 76, 1913, 164.

—— " Accidents which occurred through Colour-Blindness,"
Lancet, 181, 1911, 879–80.

—— " The Relation of Light Perception to Colour Perception," *Proc. Royal Soc.*, B82, 1910, 458–67.

—— " The Discrimination of Colours," *Proc. Royal Soc.*,
B84, 1911, 116–7.

—— " Trichromic Vision and Anomalous Trichromatism,"
Proc. Royal Soc., 1913, 686.

—— " The Necessity for the Use of Colour Names in a Test
for Colour-Blindness," *Brit. Med. Journ.*, 2, 1912,
111–3.

—— " A Case of Colour-Blindness," *Lancet*, 182, 1912,
1684–5.

—— " New Facts of Colour-Vision," *Nature*, Aug. 25th,
1921.

Edridge-Green, F. W., *The Physiology of Vision*, London, 1921.

—— *The Physiology of Form and Colour-Vision*, London.

—— *Colour-Blindness and Colour Perception*, Int. Scientific Series, London, 1891.

—— *Hunterian Lectures on Colour-Vision and Colour-Blindness*, London, 1911.

Favre, A., *Réforme des Employés de Chemin de Fer affectés de Daltonisme*, Lyons, 1873.

—— *Recherches cliniques sur le Daltonisme*, Lyons, 1874.

Ferree, C. E., and Rand, G., "Some Areas of Colour-Blindness of an Unusual Type in the Peripheral Retina," *Journ. of Exp. Psych.*, Vol. II, 1917, 295–303.

Fick, A., *Farbenblindheit, Pflüger's Archiv*, 64, 1878.

—— *Hermann's Handbuch der Physiologie der Sinnesorgane*, Vol. III, Part 1, 1879.

Galloway, A. B., "Notes on an Interesting Case of Colour-Blindness," *Brit. Med. Journ.*, 1, 1912, 949–50.

Galton, F., *Enquiries into Human Faculty*, Everyman Library.

Goethe, J. W., *Farbenlehre*, Translation by Eastlake, London, 1840.

Gray, J., "Colour-Blind Face and Voice," *Brit. Med. Journ.*, 1, 1911, 55.

Greenwood, M., *Physiology of the Special Senses*, London, 1910.

Hall, S., "Mesmerism," *Lancet*, 1, 1845.

—— *Amer. Acad. Science and Art*, 13, 1878, 402.

Hayes, S., *American Journ. of Psych.*, 1911.

—— "Colour Defects," *Psych. Bull.*, 1910–3.

—— *Psych. Bull.*, 1915–9.

Helmholtz, H. L. F. v., "On the Theory of Compound Colours," *Phil. Mag.*, 1852.

—— *Handbuch der physiologischen Optik*, Leipzig, 1867. 2nd Ed.

—— French Translation by Javal and Klein, Paris, 1867.

Henmon, V. A. C., "The Detection of Colour-Blindness," *Journ. of Phil. Psych. and Scientific Method*, 1906, 341–4.

Henry, W. C., *Memoirs of the Life and Scientific Researches of John Dalton*, 1854.

Hering, E., *Lotos (Neue Folge)*, 6, 1885.

—— *Zur Lehre vom Lichtsinne*, Wien, 1878.

Hering, E., *Zur Erklärung der Farbenblindheit aus der Theorie der Gegenfarben*, 1880. (Reprint from *Lotos*, N.F. I, 1880.)
—— " Zur Diagnostik der Farbenblindheit," *v. Graefe's Archiv*, 36, 1890, I, 217–33.
—— " Untersuchung eines total Farbenblinden," *Pflüger's Archiv*, 49, 1891, 563–608.
—— *Grundzüge der Lehre vom Lichtsinne*, 1905.
Herschel, J. F. W., " Remarks on Colour-Blindness," *Philosophical Magazine*, 19, 1859, 148–58.
—— " Remarks on Colour-Blindness," *Proc. Royal Soc.*, 10, 1859, 72.
Hess, C., " Untersuchung eines Falles von halbseitiger Farbensinnstörung am linken Auge," *Graefe's Archiv*, 36, 1890, 3, 24–36.
—— *Archiv für Anatomie u. Physiologie*, 56, 1908, 29.
Hess u. Hering, *Pflüger's Archiv*, 71, 1898.
Hippel, v. " Ein Fall von einseitiger congenitaler Rothgrünblindheit bei normalem Farbensinn des anderen Auges," *Graefe's Archiv*, 26, 1880, part 2.
Holmgren, F., " How do the Colour-Blind see the Different Colours ? " *Proc. Royal Soc.*, 31, 1881, 302–6.
—— *Colour-Blindness in its Relation to Accidents by Rail and Sea*, Trans. by M. L. Duncan, *Smithsonian Report*, 1877, 131–95.
—— *Colour-Blindness and the Young-Helmholtz Theory of Colour*, 1871.
—— *On Forster's Perimeter and the Topography of the Colour Sense*, 1871.
—— *On Theories of Colour-Blindness*, 1873.
—— *On the Theory and Diagnosis of Colour-Blindness* 1874.
—— *De la Cécité des Couleurs dans ses Rapports avec les Chemins de Fer et la Marine*, Stockholm, 1877.
Houston, R. A., *Proc. Royal Soc. Edin.*, 42, 1922.
Howell, W. H., *A Text-book of Physiology*, 8th Ed., Philadelphia, 1909.
Huddart, J., " An Account of Persons who could not distinguish Colours," *Phil. Trans.*, 67, 1777, 260–65.
Hunter, H., *General Psychology*, Univ. of Chicago Press, 1919.
Jeffries, J., " Dangers from Colour-Blindness in Railroad Employees and Pilots," *9th Annual Report Mass. State Board of Health*, 1878.

Jeffries, J., *Colour-Blindness: its Dangers and its Detection*, Boston, 1879.

Jennings, J. E., *Colour-Vision and Colour-Blindness*, Philadelphia, 1896.

Kirschmann, A., " Some Effects of Contrast," *Amer. Journ. of Psych.*, 4, 1892, 542–57.

Kirschmann, A., " Beiträge zur Kenntniss der Farbenblindheit," *Philos. Studien*, 8, 1892–3, 173–230, 407–30.

Köllner, H., " Zur Entstehung der erworbenen Rot-Grün-Blindheit," *Zeitchs. für Sinnesphys*, 1910, 269–292.

König, A., " The Modern Development of Thomas Young's Theory of Colour-Vision," *Brit. Assoc. Report*, 1886, 431–9.

—— *Sitzungsber. der Akad. der Wissensch.*, 1897 (Blue-Yellow).

—— " Zur Kenntniss dichromatischer Farbensysteme," *Graefe's Archiv für Ophth.*, 30, 1884, part 2.

König, A., Dieterici C., " Die Grundempfindungen in normalen und anomalen Farbensystemen und ihre Intensitätsverteilung im Spektrum," *Zeitschr. für Psych. u. Physiol. der Sinnesorg.*, 4, 1892, 241–347.

Kries, v., *Nagel's Handbuch der Physiologie des Menschen.* Vol. 3, 1905. *Abhandlungen zur Physiologie der Gesichtsempfindungen.* Leipzig, 1897.

Ladd-Franklin, C., " Vision," *Baldwin's Dict. of Phil. and Psych.*, 2, 765–99.

—— *Nature*, 48, 1893, 817.

—— *Mind*, N.S., 2, 1893, 473.

—— *Psychological Rev.*, 2, 70 ; 3, 72 ; 5, 332, 503 ; 6, 82.

Ladd, G. T., and Woodworth, R. S., *Elements of Physiological Psychology*, 1911.

Leber, T., *Zehender's Klinische Monatsblätter für Augenheilkunde.* Vol. 2, 1873.

Lickley, J. D., *Physiology of the Nervous System*, 8th Ed., London, 1920.

McDougall, W., " New Observations in Support of the Young-Helmholtz Theory of Light and Colour-Vision," *Mind*, N.S., 10, 210–347.

—— *Brain*, 24, 1901, 577 ; 26, 1903, 153.

Maxwell, J. Clerk, *Trans. of Royal Soc. of Edin.*, 21, 1855, 275–297.

—— *Proc. of Royal Soc. of Edin.*, Vol. III, 299–301.

—— *Phil. Mag.*, 14, 40–47, 1857.

Maxwell, J., *Brit. Assoc. Report*, 1856.

Meyer, M. F., " An Exceedingly Rare but Typical Case of Colour-Blindness," *Psych. Bull.*, 1916.

Müller, G. E., *Zeitschr. für Psych. u. Physiol. der Sinnesorg.*, 10, 1896 ; 14, 1897.

Myers, C. S., *Experimental Psychology*, 2nd Ed., Camb. Univ. Press.

—— *Brit. Journ. of Psych.*, 2, 1908, 361.

Nagel, A., *Der Farbensinn*, 1869, Berlin.

—— Virchow and Holtzendorff's *Sammlung wissenschaftlicher Vorträge*.

Nagel, W., See Chapters in Helmholtz's *Handbuch der Physiologischen Optik*, 3rd Edition, Vol. II, 1911.

Nettleship, " Some Unusual Pedigrees of Colour-Blindness," *Trans. Ophth. Soc.*, 32, 1912, 309–36.

—— *Trans. Ophth. Soc.*, 28, 1908, 248.

Nichols, E. L., " On the Sensitiveness of the Eye to Colours of a Low Degree of Saturation," *Amer. Journ. of Science and Arts*, Series 3, 30, 1885, 37–41.

Parsons, J. H., *An Introduction to the Study of Colour-Vision*, 2nd Ed., Camb. Univ. Press.

—— *Manual of Diseases of the Eye*, 2nd Ed., 1912.

—— *Pathology of the Eye*, 1908.

—— " Critical Review," *Brit. Journ. of Ophth.*, 1922, July, Aug., Sept.

Peddie, W., *Colour-Vision*, 1922.

—— " Note on Some Generally Accepted Views regarding Vision," *Proc. Royal Soc. Edin.*, 25, pt. 2, 1904–5.

—— " On a Case of Colour-Blindness," *Trans. Royal Soc. Edin.*, 38, pt 2.

Pole, W., *Trans. Royal Soc.*, 149, 1859, 323.

—— *Proc. Royal Soc.*, 1856.

—— *Trans. Royal Soc., Edin.*, 1893, also *Proc.* 1893.

—— " Colour-Blindness," *Nature*, 1879.

—— " Further Data on Colour-Blindness," *Phil. Mag. Series*, 5, 35, 1892.

—— " Article on Helmholtz," *Phil. Mag. Series*, 5, 35, 1893.

—— " Article on Hering," *Phil. Mag. Series*, 5, 36, 1893.

Pryn, W. W., " Tests for Colour-Vision," *Brit. Med. Journ.*, 2, 1910.

Raehlmann, " Beiträge zur Lehre vom Daltonismus und seiner Bedeutung für die Young'sche Farbentheorie." *Graefe's Archiv für Ophth.*, 19, 1873.

Ramsay, " On Colour-Blindness," *Bristol Nat. Soc. Proc.*, 5, 1886–7.

Rayleigh, Lord, " Colour Equations," *Nature*, 25, 1881–2, 64–6.

Report of the Departmental Committee on Sight Tests, London, 1912.

Report of Committee on Colour-Vision, Proc. Royal Soc., 51, 1892.

Richardson, F., " An Unusual Case of Colour-Blindness," *Psych. Bull.*, 8, 1911. American Journal of Psychology, 34, 1923.

Roaf, H. E., *Journ. of Physiology*, 57, 1923.

—— *Quarterly Journ. of Exper. Phys.*, 14, 1924.

Rivers, W. H. R., " Vision " in Schäfer's *Text-book of Physiology*, 2, 1900.

—— *Memorandum to Departmental Committee, Minutes of Evidence*, 1912.

Rood, O. N., *A Student's Text-book of Colour*, New York, 1881.

Sanford, E. C., *Experimental Psychology*, Boston, 1903.

Schufelt, S. W., " A Case of Daltonism Affecting One Eye," *New York Med. Rev.*, 23, 1883.

Schumann, F., " Ein ungewöhnlicher Fall von Farbenblindheit." *Bericht der I. Kong. für exp. Psy.*, 1904, 10–13.

Schuster, " Experiments with Lord Rayleigh's Colour Box," *Proc. Royal Soc.*, 48, 1890, 140–9.

Seebeck, A. v., " Ueber den bei manchen Personen vorkommenden Mangel an Farbensinn," *Poggendorff's Annalen der Physik und Chemie*, 42, 1837, 177.

Sherrington, C. S., *Physiological Abstracts*, 5, 161.

Spurzheim, J. G., *Phrenology*, 1825.

Stilling, J., Lehre von den Farbenempfindungen, *Klin. Monatsblatt*, 1873.

—— *Prüfung des Farbensinnes*, Cassel, 1877.

—— " Ueber Entstehung und Wesen der Anomalien des Farbensinnes," *Zeitschr. für Sinnesphys.*, 1910.

Taylor, G. H., " Congenital Colour-Blindness," *Brit. Med. Journ.*, 2, 1910, 437.

Thomson,W., and Weiland, C., *Detection of Colour-Blindness. Norris and Oliver's System of Diseases of the Eye*, Vol. II, 315–52.

Titchener, E. B., *A Text-book of Psychology*.

Tschermak, A., *Ueber Kontrast und Irradiation, Ergebnisse der Physiol.*, 1903, 726–98.

Usher, C. H., " A Pedigree of Colour-Blindness," *Trans. Ophth. Soc.*, 32, 1912, 352–61.

Warren, H. C., *Human Psychology.*

Watson, *Proc. Royal Soc.*, 1913, pt. 3.

Whipple, G. M., *Manual of Mental and Physical Tests*, Vol. 1, Baltimore, 1914. 2nd Edition.

Whitmell, C. T., *Colour.*

Williams, M. C., *Description of an Unusual Case of Partial Colour-Blindness*, Psych. Monograph, 25, 1918.

Wilson, G., *Researches on Colour-Blindness*, Edin., 1855.

Witmer, I.., *Analytical Psychology*, London, 1902.

Woodworth, R. S., *Psychology: A Study of Mental Life*, London, 1921.

Young, T., *Lectures on Natural Philosophy*, 2, 315, 1807.

—— *Phil. Trans.*, 1801, pt. 1, p. 33.

INDEX

Abney : 2, 4, 14, 17, 19, 26, 45, 57, 63, 71, 72
achromatopia : 21
acquired colour-blindness : 9, 25*ff*
after-images : 142, 145*f*, 186, 190, 192, 194, 199, 201, 202, 214
Aitken : 35
Ångström unit : 111
anomalous trichromate : 13, 14, 15, 29, 44, 57, 63, 110, 125, 147, 196, 205*ff*
artificial colour-blindness : 30
atmospheric conditions, effect of : 167*ff*, 171

Biedermann : 45
blue-blindness : 18
blue-yellow blindness : 12, 17*ff*, 59*f*
Board of Trade : 14
Boll : 54
Bradley colours : 96, 105, 116*ff*, 138, 140, 142, 186, 190, 192, 194, 196, 202, 205, 206, 214
Burch, G. J. : 30

central scotoma : 16, 21, 25
Chevreul chromatic circle : 23
Clerk-Maxwell : 7, 8, 9, 18, 95, 224
Collins : 16
colour discs : 8
colour equations : 8, 20*f*, 95*ff*, 175, 186, 195, 197, 203
colour-filter hypothesis : 181
colour mixing : 95, 192, 194, 195, 199, 201, 202, 204, 206, 207
colour naming : 74*ff*, 199, 203, 205
colour preference : 183
coloured picture : 182
colour screen : 172
coloured shadows : 141, 142*ff*, 186, 190, 192, 194, 195, 197, 199, 201, 202, 204, 206
colour theories : 1, 31*ff*
colour triangle : 137
colour weakness : 13
complementary colours : 41
constancy of colours : 214

contrast experiments : 141*ff*, 186 ; rings contrast : 142, 144*f*, 186, 190, 192, 194, 195, 197, 199, 201, 202, 206 ; effect of : 164*f*, 214

Dalton : 4, 5, 6, 7, 75
Daltonism : 4, 5
dangerous colour-blind : 167, 171
Dawbeney : 22
deuteranope : 6, 12, 16, 17, 19, 45, 52
dichromate, dichromic : 2, 14, 15, 17, 35, 56, 57, 111, 209
dichromasy, dichromatism : 10, 14, 16, 17, 20, 65, 80, 202, 211
Donders : 19, 22, 23, 209
Drever : 116
duplicity theory : 37, 53

Earle, Pliny : 223
Ebbinghaus : 53
Edridge-Green : 14*ff*, 27, 54, 55, 57, 72, 74, 76, 136, 140, 141, 159, 165, 167, 169, 195, 215, 216, 223
Edridge-Green theory : 53*ff*, 215, 218
Edridge-Green lantern : 15, 16, 139, 153*ff*, 187, 190, 194, 196, 199, 201, 205, 207, 208, 214

Ferree : 146
Festing : 57
Fick : 35
foveal blindness : 23, 24, 25
Fraunhofer lines : 111

Goethe : 5
green-blind : 2, 4, 9, 11, 33, 34, 37, 47, 72, 97, 98, 146, 217, 218, 219
greenish red, *vide* reddish green
Greenwood : 20, 30
ground glass : 167
Guttman : 13

Harris : 3, 4, 22
Hayes : 1, 16, 17, 63, 74, 110, 111, 184, 218, 225

235

Helmholtz : 3, 8, 11, 12, 13, 14, 31, 35, 36, 100, 218, 224 ; theory, *vide* Young-Helmholtz
heptachromic : 57
heredity : 218, 223, 224
Hering : 11, 12, 14, 19, 20, 23, 24, 40, 41, 42, 44, 45, 46, 219
Hering theory : 11, 37, 40*ff*, 219, 220
Herschel : 6
Hess : 17, 22, 23, 24, 44
hexachromic : 57
Hill, Leonard : 20
v. Hippel : 9, 10, 16
Holmgren : 2, 7, 9, 10, 19, 33, 34, 61, 71, 72, 73, 75
Holmgren wool test : 2, 9, 10, 61*ff*, 77, 107, 176, 186, 190, 191, 193, 196, 198, 203, 206, 223 ; results : 64*ff*, 82 ; naming : 86*ff*, 139, 140
Horner's Law : 224
Houston : 217, 224, 225
Huddart : 3

Jeffries, Joy : 2, 22, 27, 73, 75, 76, 222

Köllner : 29
König : 19, 24, 25, 35
v. Kries : 10, 12, 13, 19, 24, 37, 45, 53
Kühne : 24, 54

Ladd-Franklin, C. : 24, 47, 50, 53, 190, 218
Ladd-Franklin theory : 47*ff*, 51, 217, 220
Leber : 35

Marshall, Devereux : 54
Maxwell, *vide* Clerk
McDougall : 37, 218
McDougall's Theory : 37*ff*
mineral pigments : 7
monochromat : 20, 38, 215, 216
monocular colour-blindness : 9, 10, 16
Müller, G. E. : 46*f*
Myers : 100

Nagel : 13, 17
Nagel cards : 79, 147*ff*, 187, 190, 192, 194, 195, 197, 199, 201, 202, 205

Nettleship : 54
neutral band : 36, 37, 97, 114, 115, 120, 121, 125, 129, 130, 131, 134, 135, 138, 140, 141, 173, 191, 192, 195, 198, 200, 202, 204, 210, 213, 216, 219 ; extra spectral : 120, 122, 123, 125*f*, 127, 135, 136, 138, 141, 213, 216, 219
neutral glasses : 166*f*
neutral point : 19, 20
Newton : 209
Nichols : 6
nomenclature : 74*ff*, 107, 195, 197, 199, 202
Norris and Oliver : 36, 37, 222
nystagmus : 20, 21, 25

organic dyes : 7

painting test : 171*ff*
Parsons : 17, 20, 22, 111
partial colour-blindness : 12, 17, 18, 19, 33
Peddie : 137, 138, 140, 141, 219
pentachromic : 57
percentage : 220*ff*
photerythrous : 12, 45
photochemical substance : 24, 31, 55
photometer, v. Hippel : 10
photophobia : 20
Pole : 9, 11, 12, 75, 208, 209
Priestley, Rev. J. : 3
protanope : 6, 12, 16, 17, 19, 45, 53
Prussian blue : 7
Purkinje phenomenon : 12

Raehlmann : 114
Rand : 146
Rayleigh : 13
Rayleigh's equation : 109*ff*, 120, 125, 195, 196, 205, 206
red-anomalous : 102, 206
red-blind : 2, 9, 11, 30, 33*f*, 36, 47, 51, 72, 98, 132, 217, 218, 219
reddish-green : 40, 85, 87, 88, 89, 90, 91, 92, 93, 113, 114, 121, 122, 123, 128, 129, 136*ff*, 165, 194
red-green blindness : 3*ff*, 19, 43*ff*, 47, 50, 52, 59*f*, 63, 86, 109, 191
ribbed glass : 168
Richardson : 17
Richarz : 52

INDEX

237

T - #0609 - 101024 - C0 - 216/138/0 - PB - 9781138953116 - Gloss Lamination